PROCEEDINGS OF THE ACADEMY OF KYUNGRAK OF THE DPRK

KYUNGRAK SYSTEM
AND
THEORY OF SANAL

These two papers were read by Professor Kim Bong Han at the first scientific symposium of the Korean Society of Kyungrak held in Pyongyang on April 15, 1965

1965 No.2

CuriousPages Publishing
Bristol, United Kingdom

First published 1965 by the Medical Science Press, Pyongyang, Korea.

This edition published 2016 by CuriousPages Publishing, Bristol, United Kingdom

ISBN 978-0-9957703-3-1 (full colour edition)
ISBN 978-0-9957703-7-9 (black and white edition)

Editorial preface

For thousands of years, the paths of the acupuncture meridians had been known, but until the 1960's no anatomical structures could be found that corresponded to the meridians. In 1962, Bong-Han Kim (born 1916), a North Korean medical surgeon at Pyongyang Medical University, published the first scientific evidence of these structures. He was then appointed director of the North Korean National *Academy of Kyung-Rak* ("Kyung-Rak" is the Korean term for "meridian"). And up until 1965, he produced four further articles detailing his extensive research into these structures. His findings were detailed most thoroughly in his last two reports, of 1963 and (the current book) 1965, which were both translated into English.

However, his reports did not describe the methods and materials necessary for his experiments to be duplicated. In particular, the new anatomical vessels he identified were extremely fine, almost transparent and required the use of a specific blue dye to render them visible under a microscope.

In 1967, S. Fujiwara, a Japanese anatomy professor, was able to reproduce some of Kim's results (locating these new vessels inside blood vessels and on the surfaces of organs), but later recalled that it took him about half a year of hard work to obtain these limited results.

Kim's reports described a range of completely new anatomical structures, including node-like structures at the acupoints, connected with fine vessels, which extended to the internal organs, and also existed within blood and lymph vessels and throughout the nervous system. These structures were reported to circulate embryonic-like cells which transformed into the various cells required by our body's organs and tissues, and which were circulated in this "meridian" system to complete their transformation. And the purpose of the entire system was said to be the continuous repair and regeneration of key cells in our organs and elsewhere.

However, these astonishing claims were then neglected worldwide until the year 2000, when Kwang-Sup Soh, a physics professor at Seoul National University (SNU), set up a team to investigate Kim's finding. The team soon successfully confirmed the presence of these new vessels inside the blood vessels of rabbits but experienced problems in reproducing their results. They realized they needed the assistance of a skilful researcher in microsurgery and optical imaging due to the extremely small size and the semitransparent nature of these new vessels, so the team visited Professor Fujiwara in Osaka, who provided a video of the experimental procedures he developed in the 1960's.

This enabled the SNU team to reproduce Fujiwara's results and they identified these new vessels floating within blood vessels, on the surface of rabbit intestines and the bladder, on the surface of a rabbit's liver, floating inside lymph vessels, in the bovine heart, in rat brain, spinal cord and nerves. And it has also been confirmed that the fluid circulated within these vessels is abundant with immune cells such as macrophages and mast cells; and also contain very small embryonic cells, similar to stem cells.

To date, every one of Kim's procedures that have been reproduced have confirmed his claims. However the scope of his work was tremendous, and many aspects of it have still not been investigated or reproduced by other researchers. Perhaps most significantly, there has been great difficulty in identifying the vessels which Kim found running through our skin (which are said to correspond with the meridians), a task that poses even greater technical difficulties than identifying the vessels elsewhere in our body.

The termination of Bong-Han Kim's research

Near the start of his research in 1962, the North Korean leadership awarded Bong-Han Kim the People's Prize for his work, and even honoured him by representing him on a postage stamp.

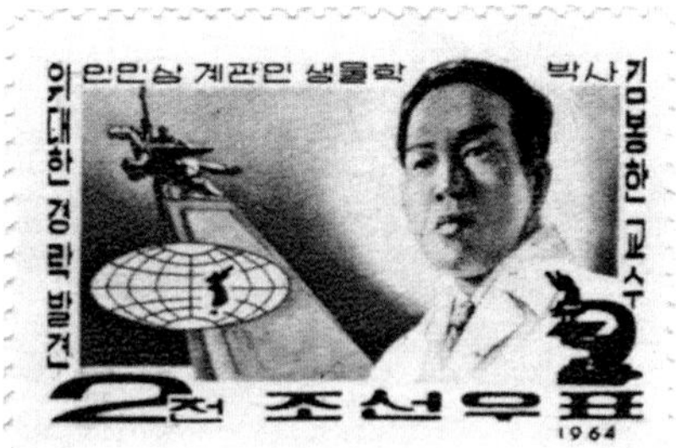

But not long after the publication of the current book (in 1965), the Kyung-Rak Institute was inexplicably closed and Kim was not heard of again.

At the time, North Korea was experiencing great economic difficulties and political uncertainty, with its leadership changing allegiances between the socialist superpowers, China, Russia and East Germany. Added to this, Kim's findings were at odds with conventional biology, and the second half of his last book was even more scientifically controversial, with Kim himself stating, "The theory of [*p-microcell*], of course, requires the re-examination of the cell theory and other cardinal problems of biology".

The leadership's decision to close down his institute has to be viewed in the context of all these facts. If the controversial nature of his research *was* a factor, the recent duplication of many of his findings has certainly vindicated his work.

The current text

The current book is the complete text of Kim's 1965 book, including over 100 colour photos. The book describes his full research findings into the acupuncture meridian system and its anatomical purpose. This is an extremely important book and is a fascinating read for any serious student or practitioner of acupuncture.

The editorial policy

The source text was the 1965 English translation of the original Korean text. The source text used a mixture of English and American spellings, some idiosyncratic grammar and some obsolete medical spellings (such as "profund"). But since the text is of scientific interest, the spellings and grammar of the original English translation have been maintained in this edition. The text has been re-typeset, and for reference purposes the page numbers of the 1965 English edition are indicated thus "[p10]".

Fletcher Kovich, December 2016, Bristol, UK.

CONTENTS

KYUNGRAK SYSTEM

INTRODUCTION

In our previous reports it was pointed out that Kyungrak exists as a new anatomico-histological structure ("On the Substance of Kyungrak," Korean Medicine No. 1, 1962) and later we brought to light its existence as a system ("On the Kyungrak System," Proceedings of the Academy of Medical Sciences, D.P.R.K., No. 5, Nov. 30, 1963).

Our study for the overall clarification of the Kyungrak system has been continued. For this purpose, it was necessary to throw light on the forms and structures of its constituent parts and to study the order of their distribution. We have studied the structure of the Kyungrak system, regarding it as a system of the circulation of Bonghan liquor which particularly abounds in deoxyribonucleic acid (DNA).

Following are the subjects, upon which our efforts have been focused:

1. The forms and structures of the constituent parts of the Kyungrak system,
2. The features of distribution of its constituent parts and
3. The system of circulation of the Bonghan liquor.

Our first and foremost object was to bring to light the inner structure of the Kyungrak system so as to ascertain the essential biological significance of this system.

The results obtained in the course of our research work are presented in this treatise. [p9]

Part 1. Constituent parts of the Kyungrak System

The deep-going researches into the Kyungrak system have revealed the existence and distribution of other Bonghan ducts and corpuscles than those which have been formerly disclosed.

In the experiment, usual anatomico-histological methods were mainly employed, along with the extensive application of histo-physiological methods. Rabbits and some other animals were used in the experiment.

Observations were *also* made on man.

The constituent parts of the Kyungrak system are the Bonghan ducts and Bonghan corpuscles. Every Bonghan duct links Bonghan corpuscles together and every Bonghan corpuscle is connected with Bonghan ducts.

Chapter I. Bonghan duct

There are several kinds of Bonghan ducts.

1. The Bonghan ducts floating in the blood and lymphatic vessels are called the internal (intravascular) Bonghan ducts.

2. The Bonghan ducts distributed on the surface of the organs, independently of the blood and lymphatic vessels and nerves, are called the intra-external Bonghan ducts. [p10]

3. The Bonghan ducts running along the outer surface of the walls of blood and lymphatic vessels are called the external (extravascular) Bonghan ducts. the external Bonghan ducts sometimes run, either independently of blood vessels or along nerves.

4. The Bonghan ducts distributed in the central and the peripheral nervous system, running inside the central canal of the spinal cord and the cerebral ventricles, are called the neural Bonghan ducts.

I. General structure of Bonghan duct

The afore-said Bonghan ducts, somewhat different as they are from each other, have the following common features:

A Bonghan duct consists of a bundle of Bonghan ductules. The wall of the Bonghan ductules is formed of endothelial cells with peculiar rod shaped nuclei which are intensively stained. Besides, the Bonghan ductule has the outer membrane composed of peculiar smooth muscle-like cells, cells of outer membrane, and of fine fibers.

In the Bonghan ductule basophile granules and small nucleus-like structures are often found.

There are fibrous structures and amorphous substance between ductules. The ductules are bound up into a bundle by periductium (the surrounding membrane of the Bonghan duct). Periductium has its cells with spherical or spindle-shaped nuclei and abundant cytoplasm (Fig. 1).

II. Internal Bonghan duct

The internal Bonghan duct is found floating in the blood and lymphatic vessels. Under the stereomicroscope, the Bonghan ducts running inside the blood vessels are not to be seen from outside, while those inside the lymphatic vessels are to be observed.

The internal Bonghan duct looks, under the stereomicroscope, like a yellowish milk-white thread, and in some cases, the flow of its contents can be observed. When a blood vessel is incised, a fine Bonghan duct is found in it.

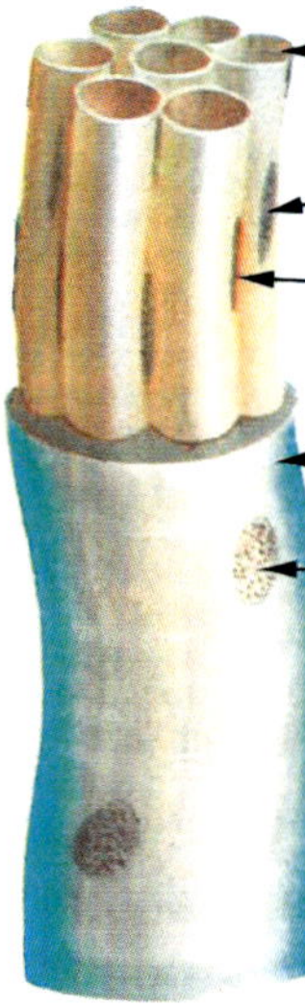

Figure 1. Diagram of the Bonghan duct

This Bonghan duct is very soft and glutinous. One or several [p11] internal Bonghan ducts may be observed in one blood vessel. These Bonghan ducts consist of bundles of several or scores of Bonghan ductules.

The calibre of the Bonghan ductule is about 5-15 microns in the fresh specimen. In some cases, the ductule is filled with so much contents that its calibre is extended to 40-50 microns. Very thin ductules with a calibre of about 1 micron are also found sometimes.

Structure of Bonghan ductule

1. Endothelial cells of Bonghan ductule

The nucleus of an endothelial cell of the Bonghan ductule takes the shape of a long rod with pointed ends. Its inner structure is hardly observed as it is deeply stained with hematoxylin. Its length reaches 15-20 microns.

The nucleus does not bulge towards the inner surface of the ductule. The space between endothelial nuclei is bigger than in the blood and lymphatic vessels (Fig. 2).

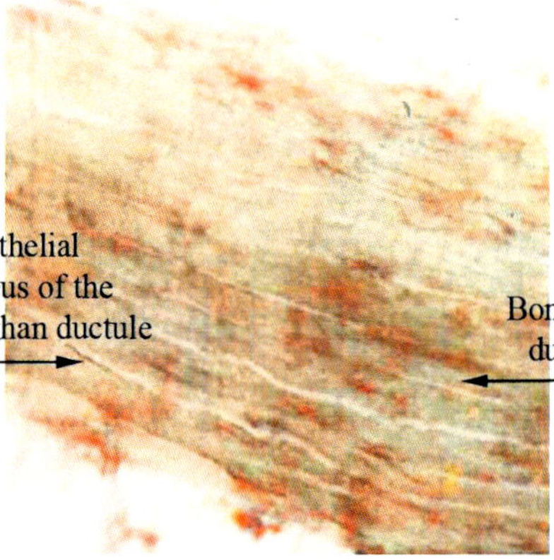

Figure 2. Internal Bonghan duct (x160)

When examined under the electron microscope, the wall of the Bonghan ductule is somewhat high in electron density and thin, about 0.1-0.2 micron, and is surrounded by fine fibrous structures.

In the wall of the Bonghan ductule long rod-shaped endothelial nuclei are found. Their properties are entirely different from those of blood or lymphatic capillaries. Their chromatin is homogeneous and electron is opaque. Nucleoli are hardly to be seen here.

The endoplasm of cytoplasm is observed at both ends of the rod-shaped nucleus and it merges into the wall of the Bonghan ductule. The boundary of cells is scarcely discernible (Fig. 3 and 4).

2. Outer membrane of Bonghan ductule

Cells of the outer membrane cover the Bonghan ductule. They are rather large spindle-shaped cells with ellipsoidal nuclei, somewhat looking like the smooth muscle cell.

In the nucleus fine chromatin granules are found and the nuclear membrane is clearly distinguished.

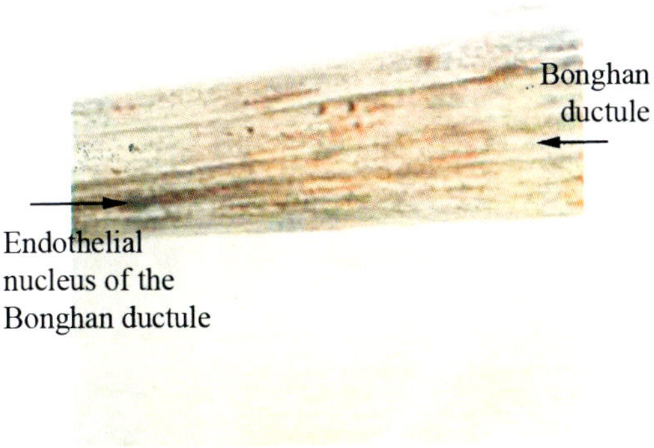

Figure 3. Internal Bonghan duct (x400)

The cell body is of an elongated-spindle shape and the nucleus is located in its centre. [12]

Fine basophile granules are found scattered in the cytoplasm.

As to the shape of the cell, it is either of an elongated spindle or oval form. This suggests that the same cell of the outer membrane assumes two appearances, since it plays the role of contractile element.

The ordinary size of the cell nucleus of the outer membrane is about 13-27 microns x 4-5 microns.

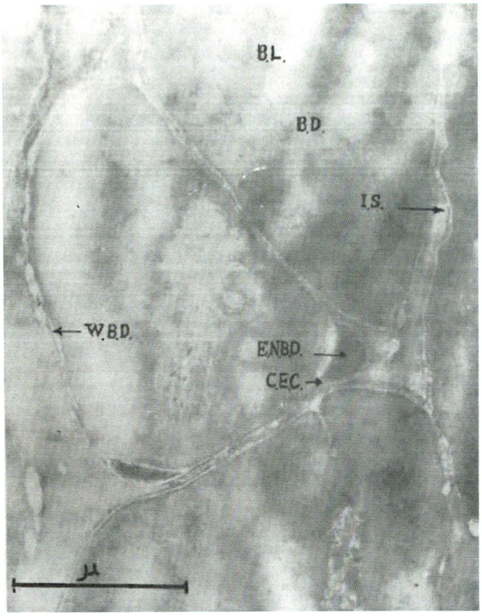

Figure 4. Electron micrograph of the internal Bonghan duct (cross section) (x42,000)

BL – Bonghan liquor
BD – Bonghan ductule
IS – Interstitial substance
WBD – Wall of Bonghan ductule
ENBD – Endothelial nucleus of the Bonghan ductule
CEC – Cytoplasm of endothelial cell

The Bonghan ductules are surrounded by fine, longitudinal and circular fibres crossing each other. These ductules often present peculiar cross-banding thanks to the circular fibres. Rather thick longitudinal fibres between the ductules are to be seen. These fibres are all argyrophile.

3. Contents of Bonghan ductule

The Bonghan ductule contains basophile granules, basophile structures of various shapes, and nucleus-like structures, which are all positive in the Feulgen reaction. But formed elements are not always seen in the Bonghan ductule (Figure 5).

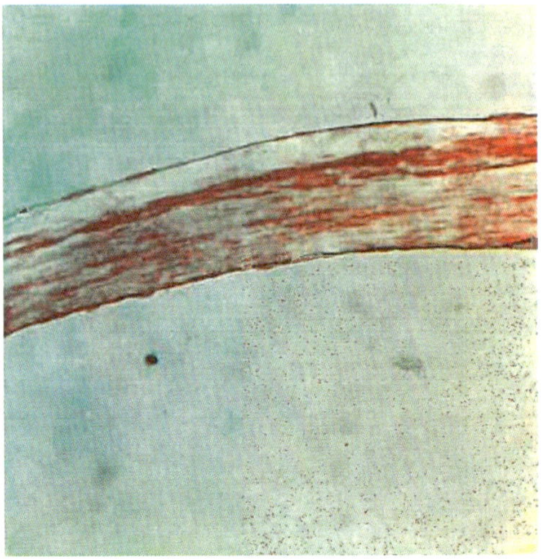

Figure 5. Internal Bonghan duct (Feulgen reaction) (x160)

Even in the same Bonghan duct some ductules may be filled with formed elements and others may not. Besides, in the Bonghan ductules, small granules positive in adrenalin reaction by Hillarp's method are often crowded here and there (Figure 6).

4. Periductium of Bonghan duct

The Bonghan ductules are bound up into a bundle by a thin periductium. The cells of the periductium are very scanty in number. They are rich in cytoplasm and their nuclei are spherical or oval ranging from 6 to 12 microns in diameter.

III. Intra-external Bonghan duct

The intra-external Bonghan ducts run freely on the surface of the internal organs in the thoracic and abdominal cavities and spread reticulately, sending out branches to various internal organs. The stereomicroscopic and microscopic findings of the intra-external Bonghan duct are not much different from those of the internal Bonghan duct. [p13]

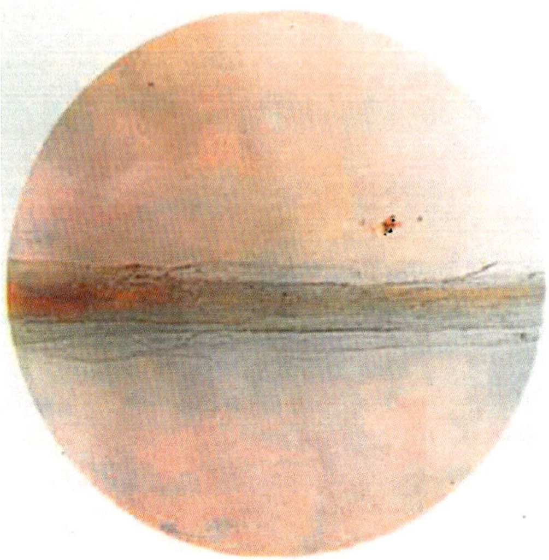

Figure 6. Internal Bonghan duct (Hillarp-Hökfelt reaction) (x400)

Examined under a stereomicroscope, the fresh specimen of intra-external Bonghan duct is ascertained as a semi-transparent, milk-white filiform structure, which is covered with a very thin and transparent connective tissue membrane. It is of somewhat harder consistency than the internal Bonghan duct. The intra-external Bonghan duct also consists of a bundle of Bonghan ductules.

Between these ductules more and thicker fibres than those of the internal Bonghan duct run longitudinally and finer fibres run obliquely or crosswise; such specific, cross-banding as in the internal Bonghan duct is sometimes observed. The intra-external Bonghan duct also has the same endothelial nuclei and cells of the outer membrane as were observed in the internal Bonghan duct (Figure 7).

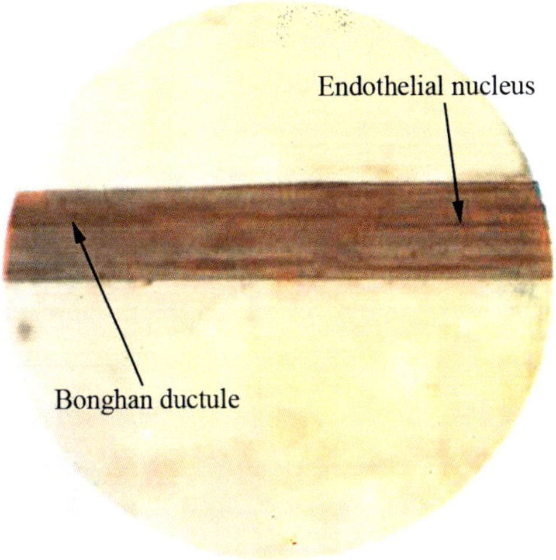

Figure 7. Intra-external Bonghan duct (x400)

The periductial cells are either spindle-shaped or oval and the structure of the nucleus is not clear. Cytoplasm is lightly stained, but the boundary of the cell is discernible.

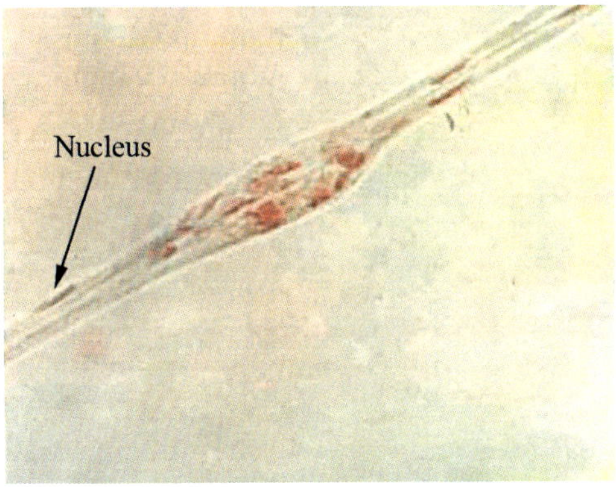

Figure 8. Intra-external Bonghan duct (Feulgen reaction) (x400)

In the periductium longitudinal fibres finer than those between ductules run obliquely and more cells of the outer membrane are seen than in the internal Bonghan ductules. The intra-external Bonghan ductules contain basophile granules, small or somewhat large, and small and spherical nucleus-like structures. All of them show positive Feulgen reaction, and the finer the granules are, the deeper the reaction is (Figure 8).

In the intra-external Bonghan ductules granules with positive adrenalin reaction are also crowded here and there. This suggests the manner of movement of the contents of the Bonghan ducts.

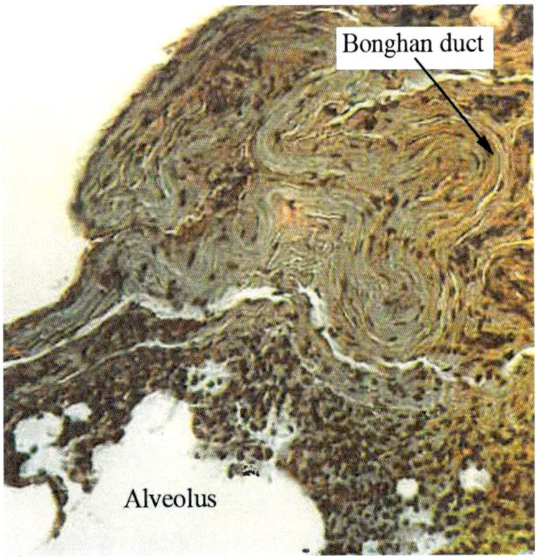

Figure 9. External Bonghan duct (in the lung) (x160)

IV. External Bonghan duct

The external Bonghan duct in the living specimen is seen as a semitransparent and somewhat yellowish structure, which is covered with connective tissue attended by abundant blood capillaries. In the external Bonghan ductule are observed mainly granules and structures of basophile character, and rarely nucleus-like structures are scattered. Other morphological features of the external ductule are similar to those of the internal Bonghan ductule (Figure 9).

The external Bonghan duct linking superficial Bonghan corpuscles with each other is called the superficial Bonghan duct. This duct penetrates into the profound layer of the corium, connecting superficial [p14] Bonghan corpuscles with each other.

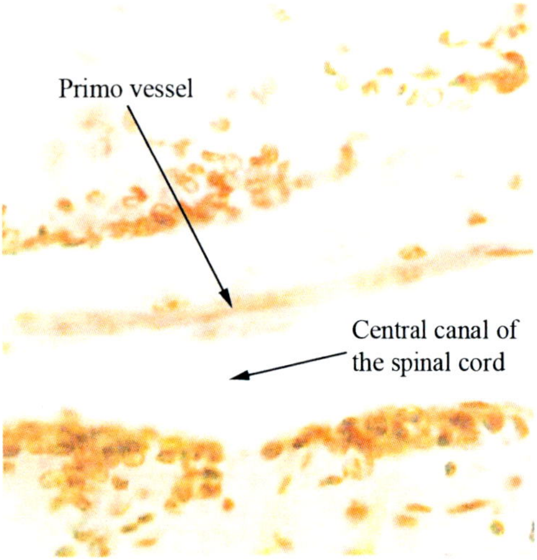

Figure 10. Neural Bonghan duct (in central conal of spinal cord) (Van Gieson stain) (x400)

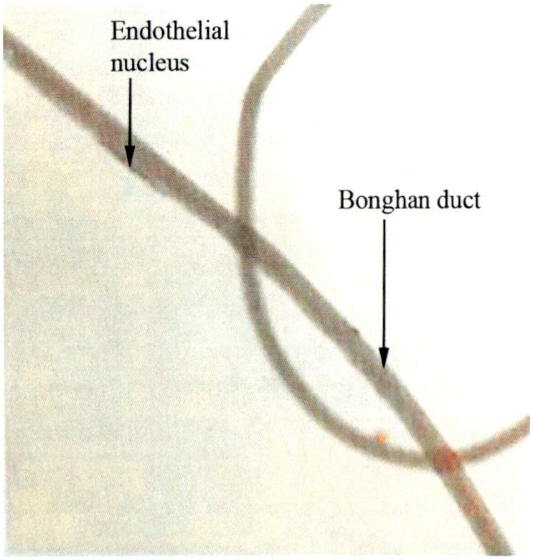

Figure 11. Neural Bonghan duct (x400)

The superficial Bonghan duct has a particular periductium which is composed of connective tissue on which blood capillaries are densely distributed. The space between the periductium and the external Bonghan duct is filled with the tissue fluid. When the superficial Bonghan duct is cut, the duct sometimes protrudes out of the periductium.

The superficial Bonghan duct sends forth so many rectangular branches into the corium as to form a net in a peculiar way.

V. Neural Bonghan duct

The neural Bonghan duct is semi-transparent, lightly milk-white in the living specimen and is of very soft consistency.

The neural Bonghan duct is a bundle of two to four Bonghan ductules and the space between endothelial nuclei is wider than in other ducts.

The neural Bonghan ductule has cells of the outer membrane with fusiform or ellipsoidal nuclei measuring 5-20 microns in size (Figure 10 and Figure 11).

Loose argyrophile fibres lie in the substance between Bonghan ductules.

The neural Bonghan ductule also contains basophile granules, basophile structures and nucleus-like structures of positive Feulgen reaction (Figure 12).

Chapter II. Bonghan corpuscle

The Bonghan corpuscles are classified into the superficial and the profund[1] Bonghan corpuscle and the latter again into the internal (intra-vascular), external (extra-vascular), intra-external, neural and intra-organic Bonghan corpuscles.

The internal Bonghan corpuscle is linked by the internal Bonghan [p15] ducts, the external corpuscle by external ducts and the superficial corpuscle by superficial ducts. The intra-external and the neural corpuscle are also linked by the ducts of relevant names respectively.

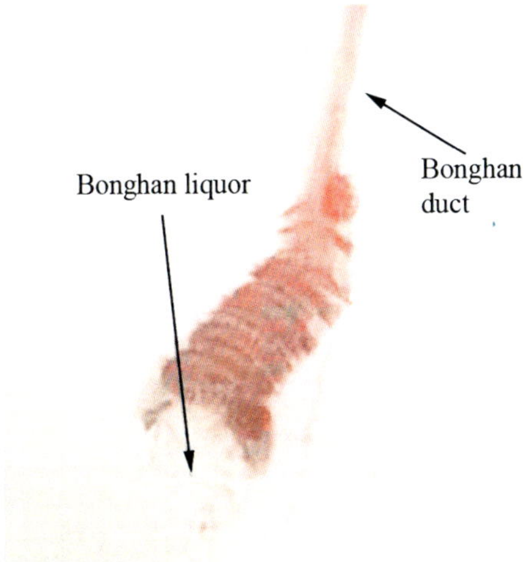

Figure 12. Neural Bonghan duct (Outflow of Bonghan liquor from the section of a Bonghan duct) (x400)

[1] An obsolete anatomical term meaning "deep within the body". Kim's original usage of this word is maintained throughout.

I. General structure of Bonghan corpuscle

A number of common features are found in the structure of the Bonghan corpuscle:

1) The basic structure of the corpuscle consists of the ramified, enlarged and anastomosed Bonghan ductules.

2) The Bonghan duct in the corpuscle contains basophile granules, small nucleus-like and somewhat large, round nucleus-like structures. Cells with pale plasm are also found and the cytoplasm often contains many chromaffine granules.

3) Reticular tissue constitutes the basis of the structure of the corpuscle.

4) The corpuscle has the outer membrane.

II. Superficial Bonghan corpuscle

1. Anatomical observations of superficial Bonghan corpuscle

The superficial Bonghan corpuscle is usually located in the corium but sometimes in the subcutaneous tissue. In most cases, its form is oval but sometimes it assumes either spindle-like or some other shapes. Very rarely, two or three corpuscles unite together to form a lobule. The size of the corpuscle varies from 0.1 to 3.0 mm in diameter, averaging from 0.5 to 1.0 mm in general.

The corpuscle is usually placed vertically to the surface of the skin, and sometimes horizontally.

The corpuscle is surrounded by loose connective tissues which are filled with rather viscous tissue fluid. And these loose connective tissues contain a dense network of blood vessels surrounding the corpuscles. These reticulated blood vessels are heavily convoluted and dilated. At the [p16] bottom of the corpuscle, the blood vessels accompanied by Bonghan ducts are connected with the corpuscle and the branches of the blood vessels surrounding the corpuscle penetrate into the corpuscle. Between the corpuscle and epidermis, part of the outer layer of the corpuscle stretches radially and its edges reach epidermis.

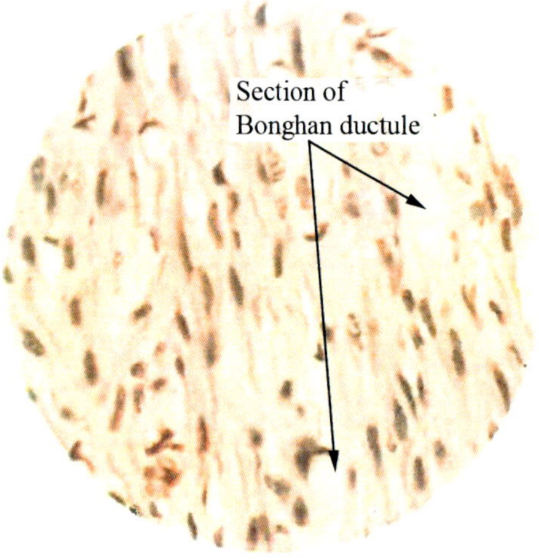

Figure 13. Bonghan ductule in the outer layer of a superficial Bonghan corpuscle (x400)

2. Histological structure of superficial Bonghan corpuscle

The superficial Bonghan corpuscle is composed of the outer layer and inner substance.

1) A striking feature in the structure of the outer layer is the abundance of smooth muscle-like cells. It is divided into the thin outer circular layer and the thick inner longitudinal layer. The former covers the outer surface of the corpuscle and is loosely linked up with the surrounding connective tissues, while the latter, running longitudinally, surrounds the inner substance of the corpuscle.

In most cases, these smooth muscle-like cells send out branches, which are interlaced in a reticular form. The ellipsoidal nucleus of a smooth muscle-like cell is oval as a whole and it is located in the centre of the cell body, and the cytoplasm surrounding it is relatively scanty.

The nuclei of the smooth muscle-like cells near the inner substance have little chromatin. The smooth muscle-like cells usually lie in the outer layer, but sometimes invade into the inner substance.

2) What is important in the outer layer is the network of Bonghan ductules encircled by smooth muscle-like cells (Figure 13).

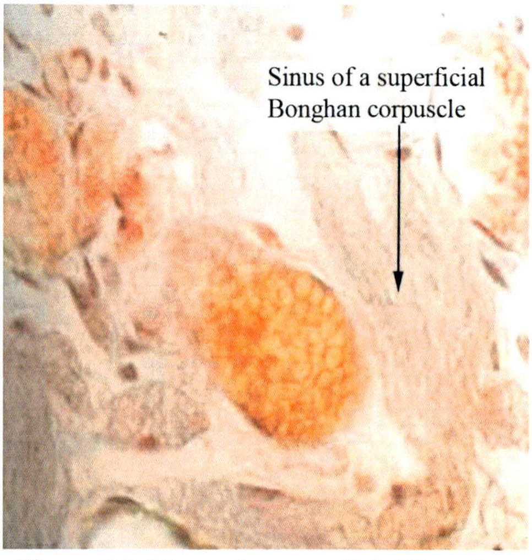

Figure 14. Sinus of a superficial Bonghan corpuscle (x400)

When a dye is injected into a point of the outer layer, it goes through the network of ductules. On longitudinal or cross sections of the specimen of the corpuscle many Bonghan ductules are seen cut crosswise or obliquely. And thin oval endothelial nuclei are also observed on their walls. The ductules contain basophile and sometimes chromaffine granules. These ductules in the outer layer are linked up with Bonghan ducts in the inner substance. The Bonghan ductules in the outer layer are surrounded spirally by argyrophile fibres, and elastic fibres in this layer run longitudinally in general. Part of the outer layer stretches into the surrounding connective tissue towards epidermis.

3) The main structures in the inner substance are tubular ones formed of enlarged Bonghan ductules which are called the sinus of the Bonghan corpuscle. [p17]

A great deal of fibrous structures are seen on the wall of the sinus. This wall is folded in a peculiar way (Figure 14).

With resorcine fuchsine, the wall of the sinus is stained deeply.

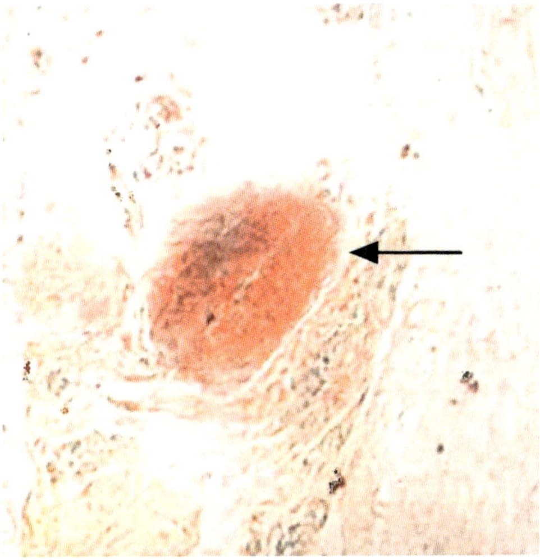

Figure 15. Sinus of a superficial Bonghan corpuscle (x160)

The sinus of the Bonghan corpuscle contains mainly basophile, Feulgen positive (Figure 15 and Figure 16) and partially, acidophile granules or chromaffine granules are mixed with them.

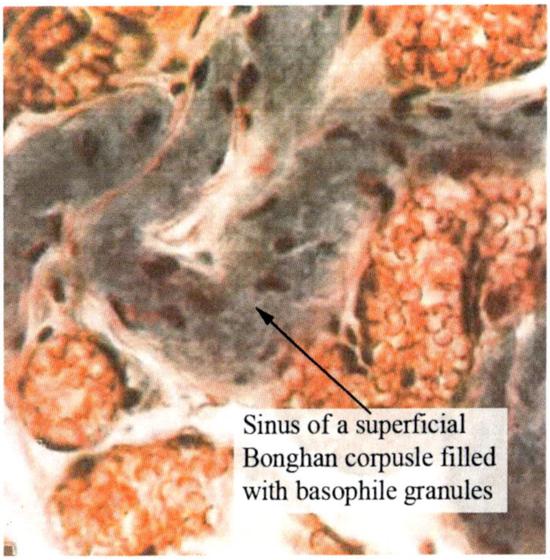

Figure 16. Sinus of a superficial Bonghan corpuscle (Verhoeff stain) (x400)

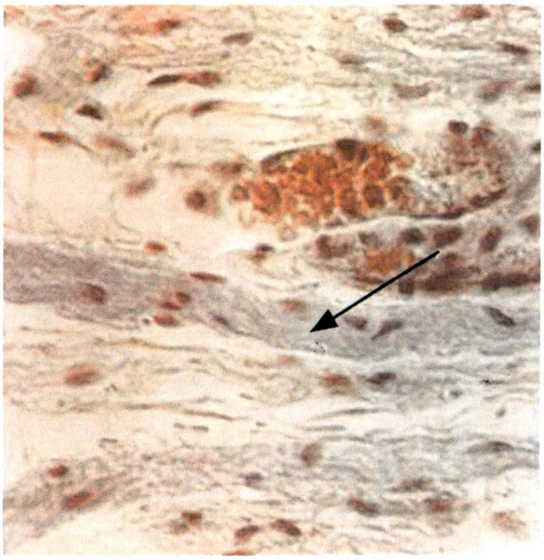

Figure 17. Sinus of a superficial Bonghan corpuscle (at the bottom of the corpuscle) (x400)

Sinuses of the superficial Bonghan corpuscles vary in their forms according to the amount of their contents. The sinus is found in the inner substance of the majority of the corpuscles and it surrounds the blood vessels there. The sinus issues slender branches which are linked with the network of Bonghan ductules in the outer layer. Sometimes, the sinus comes out through the upper part of the corpuscle and branches off. At the bottom of the corpuscle the sinus of the superficial Bonghan corpuscle meets with the external Bonghan ducts connected to the corpuscle, and with the internal Bonghan ducts inside the corpuscle (Figure 17).

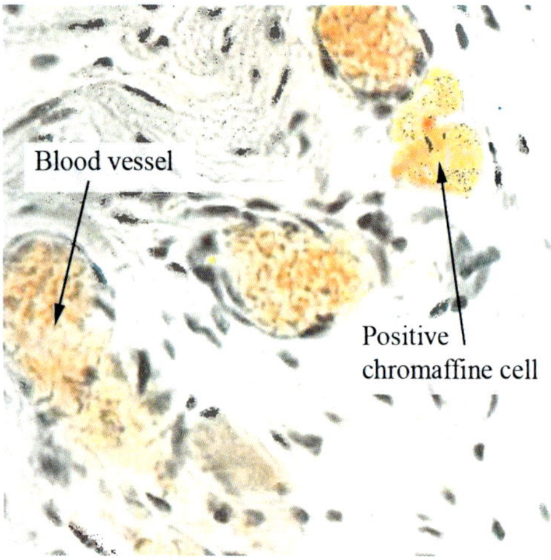

Figure 18. Superficial Bonghan corpuscle (Hillarp-Hökfelt reaction) (x400)

4) In the inner substance, mainly at its upper and middle parts, chromaffine cells form small groups near the sinus around the blood vessels. These cells are diverse in form and size, and the loci of their nuclei are also indefinite. Particularly, the contour of the cells is obscure in most cases, and sometimes, the transition of chromaffine granules to basophile granules of the sinus of the Bonghan corpuscle is observed. In certain cases, chromaffine granules are gathered together both inside and outside the sinus. These granules are positive in the Hillarp-Höckfelt and Sevki reactions (Figure 18 and Figure 19).

These granules are scattered around the blood capillaries in the inner substance of the corpuscle.

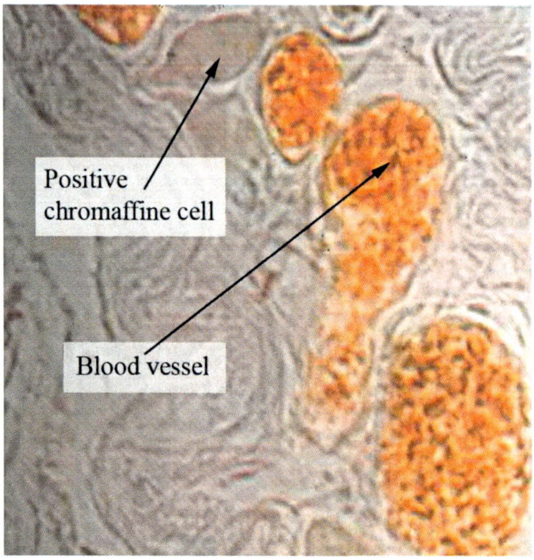

Figure 19. Superficial Bonghan corpuscle (Sevki reaction) (x400)

In the lower half of the inner substance, follicular structures formed of one or two layers of squamous or cuboidal epithelial cells can be seen. The follicular cavity contains homogeneous serous substance with very fine basophile granules.

5) The above-mentioned structures of the superficial Bonghan corpuscle are embedded in reticular tissue. Argyrophile fibres are found abundantly not only in the outer layer but also in the inner substance and they form a network there.

6) The blood vessels and nerves of the superficial Bonghan corpuscle are distributed in a peculiar way. Around the corpuscle, the network of blood vessels is particularly developed, part of which branches into the outer layer. Blood capillaries, varying

in calibre, occupy the bulk of the central part of the inner substance, heavily convoluting in a spiral form. These blood vessels, always filled with blood corpuscles, are in a very dilated state. They contain not only erythrocytes but also equally [p18] stainable granules, large and small. These blood vessels are linked with those of the outer layer and run along the bundle of vessels at the bottom of the corpuscle, finally joining the vessels outside the corpuscle. Though the nerve fibres are rather richly distributed in the tissue surrounding the Bonghan corpuscle, they are relatively scarce in the outer layer (Figure 20).

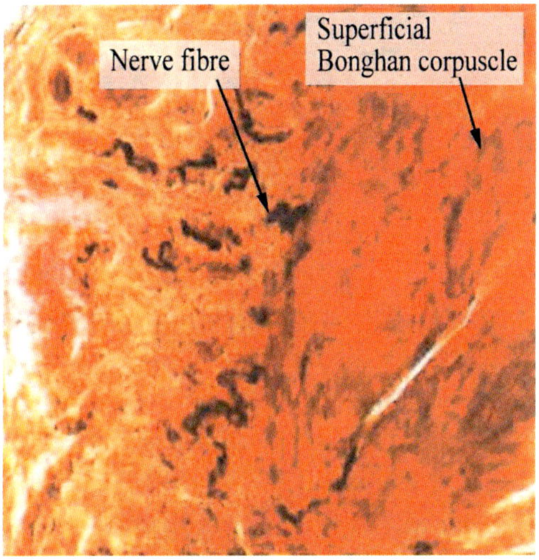

Figure 20. Nerve supply at a superficial Bonghan corpuscle (Gros-Schultze reaction) (x160)

The nerve fibres penetrating into the smooth muscle-like tissue of the outer layer terminate there, twisting spirally.

Some nerve fibres enter the inner substance through the outer layer and ramify at their terminals.

When dye solution is injected into the outer layer of the corpuscle, reticulate or heavily convoluted Bonghan ductules are noticed in the smooth muscle-like tissue. This solution, after passing through the Bonghan ductules of the outer layer, flows downwards and runs into the external Bonghan duct connected with the corpuscle and partially enters the inner substance and then flows into the internal Bonghan duct.

When the dye is injected into the inner substance of the corpuscle, it eventually runs into the internal Bonghan ducts of the blood vessels of the inner substance.

3. Electron microscopic structure of superficial Bonghan corpuscle

The nuclei of the smooth muscle-like cells have rather thin membrane and their both ends usually have irregular contour, that is, some nuclear membranes protrude and some others are indented.

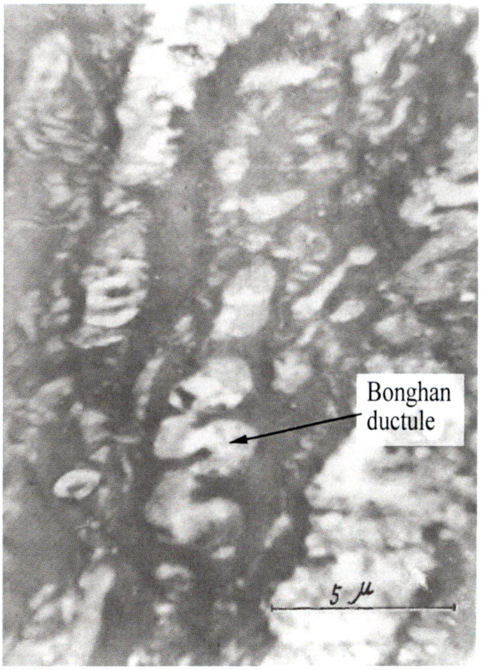

Figure 21. Electron micrograph of a Bonghan ductule in the outer layer of a superficial Bonghan corpuscle

The sarcoplasm of the smooth muscle-like cells of the outer layer adjacent to the connective tissue surrounding the corpuscle scarcely reveals its inner structure because of its extremely high electron density, but in the sarcoplasm of those bordering on the inner substance the structures of myofibrils and the endoplasmic reticulum are recognized distinctly. What is most interesting is the finding of the formation and fusion of irregular vacuolar structures at the end of the sarcoplasm. The structures thus formed contain either fine granular structures with lower electron density or irregular granular structures with higher electron density (Figure 21).

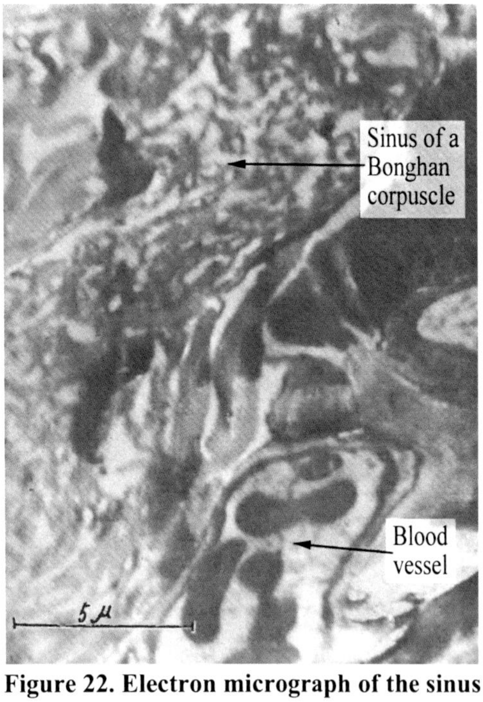

Figure 22. Electron micrograph of the sinus of a superficial Bonghan corpuscle

The thickness of the sinus wall of the superficial Bonghan corpuscle is about 0.5-1 micron and its section presents sponge-like structures, and intricately-branched septal structures and small granular structures high in electron density are found in great numbers. Chromaffine cells [p19] are filled with a lot of fine and coarse granules and many granular structures with compact electron density are mixed with them (Figure 22).

III. External Bonghan corpuscle

1. Anatomical observations of external Bonghan corpuscle

The external Bonghan corpuscles are mainly found around blood vessels.

They are easily recognized around the large blood vessels of the cervical, thoracal or abdominal regions. They are also seen around the blood vessels of medium or small calibres. The external Bonghan corpuscle is of the shape of elongated spindle and is connected at its both ends with external Bonghan ducts, and it is lightly yellow or yellowish red in living condition (Figure 23).

The surface of the corpuscle is dotted with yellow spots and is covered with a dense network of blood capillaries.

The corpuscle is lubricous on the surface and presents a clear solid appearance and it is rather easily distinguished from the surrounding tissue.

2. Histological structure of external Bonghan corpuscle

The structure of the external Bonghan corpuscle consists of Bonghan ductules and Bonghan duct sinuses, the dilated form of the former being intricately ramified and anastomosed on the base of the reticular tissues. Particularly noteworthy is the fact that besides basophile granules, nucleus-like structures and cells are crowded in the Bonghan duct sinus.

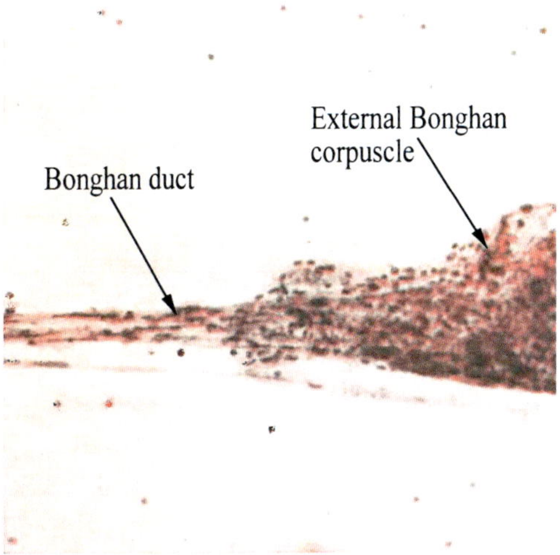

Figure 23. External Bonghan corpuscle (connected part with a Bonghan duct) (x160)

1) The Bonghan duct sinus has various cells, especially cells with pale cytoplasm and distinct chromatin structures and nuclear membrane. Chromaffine granules are also recognized sometimes (Figure 24).

These granules are positive in adrenalin reaction (Figure 25). [p20]

2) The stroma of the corpuscle is reticular tissue.

The corpuscle is covered with the outer membrane and inside it, fibrous connective tissue is found between sinuses. This connective tissue contains collagenous, elastic and argyrophile fibres.

The corpuscle is surrounded by a dense network of blood vessels, and rich blood capillaries are found between Bonghan ducts inside the corpuscle.

3) In the Bonghan ducts connected with the corpuscles, small nucleus-like structures and various basophile structures—granular, filiform, and rod-shaped, etc.—are observed.

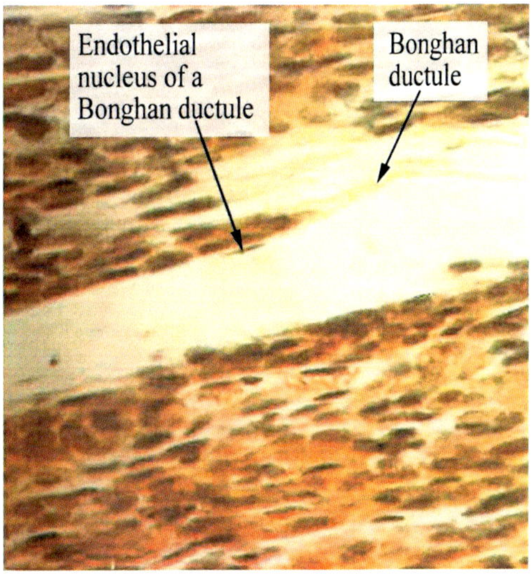

Figure 24. External Bonghan corpuscle (x400)

Figure 25. External Bonghan corpuscle (Hillarp-Hökfelt reaction) (x400)

3. Electron microscopic structure of external Bonghan corpuscle

The external Bonghan corpuscle contains cells of various shapes—spherical, elongated fusiform and irregular ones, etc. Their nuclear membranes are smooth and the chromatin particles in the nuclei are high in electron density and they lie scattered in the nuclei. Karyoplasm presents fine granular appearance and the cytoplasm of the reticular cell looks pale, since the endoplasmic reticulum and several mitochondria are located sporadically.

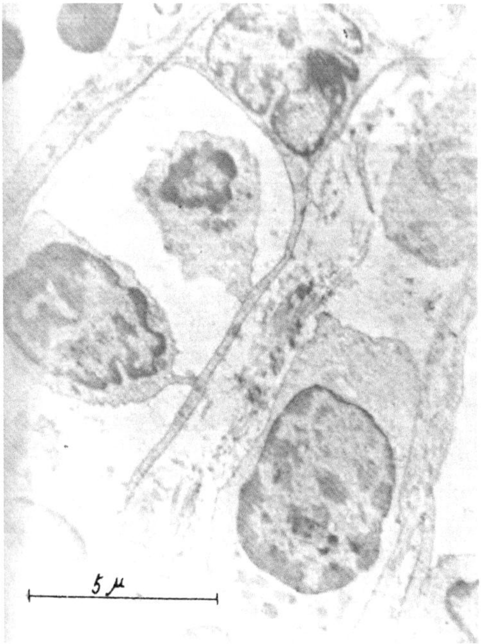

Figure 26. Electron micrograph of an external Bonghan corpuscle

The nucleus-like structures vary in shape-some are round and others irregular, and their membranes are smooth.

In the cytoplasm of some spherical cells, flat and rough surfaced endoplasmic reticula are well developed; they are arranged concentrically around the nucleus and mitochondria.

In the cytoplasm of the pale-looking cell of the external corpuscle, a nucleus or two are located in the centre or periphery of the body. These nuclei have thin membranes and rich chromatin, and the nucleoli are found in the centre of the nuclei.

The nuclear membrane sometimes is wrinkled. The periphery of the cell body is smooth or has processes sometimes. In the cytoplasm there are many vacuolar structures. The light cytoplasm of some cells contains vesicular endoplasmic reticulum and many small spherical granules higher in electron density than proper cytoplasm. But such granules can not be seen in the vacuoles. Mitochondria of an oval shape are found in a part of cytoplasm. Adjacent cells adhere closely to one another or are connected with each other through small cytoplasmic processes. Here granules of less electron density than those of the cytoplasm are gathered together.

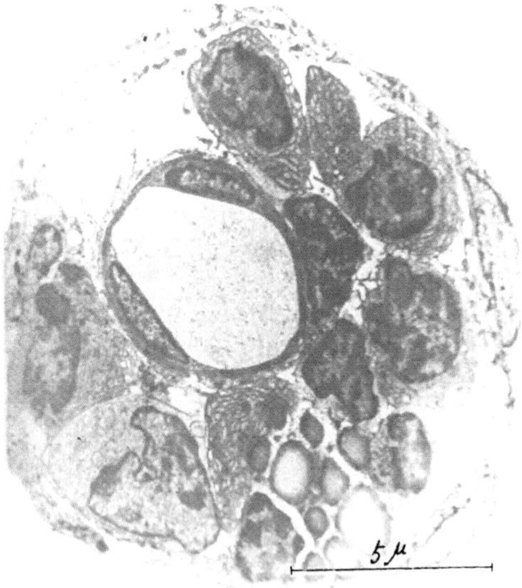

Figure 27. Electron micrograph of an external Bonghan corpuscle

Among these granules irregular spaces can be seen, where small [p21] nucleus-like structures are located and fine reticulate structures run transversely (Figure 26 - Figure 28).

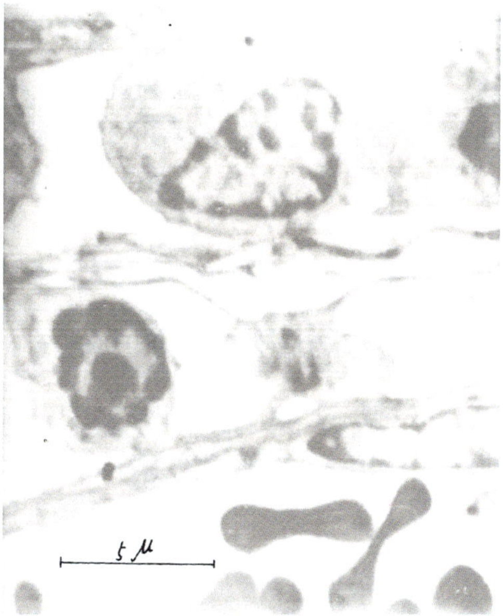

Figure 28. Electron micrograph of an external Bonghan corpuscle

IV. Internal Bonghan corpuscle

1. Anatomical observations of internal Bonghan corpuscle

The corpuscles connected by the internal Bonghan ducts in blood and lymphatic vessels are called the internal Bonghan corpuscles. These corpuscles in the vessels do not stick to their walls but float in the blood current as in the case of the internal Bonghan duct.

The internal Bonghan corpuscle looks more compact than the Bonghan duct linked with it and it is oval or spherical and usually 0.1-0.2 mm in size. It looks colourless and semi-transparent or slightly yellowish or lightly reddish. It is of soft consistency and clearly presents solid appearance. The corpuscle looks like a filled sac and its surface is usually smooth (Figure 29).

2. Histological structure of internal Bonghan corpuscle

The internal Bonghan corpuscle has peculiar cell elements.

1) The corpuscle appears as ramified and anastomosed Bonghan ductules embedded in the reticular tissue. Some ductules run through the corpuscle without sending off branches.

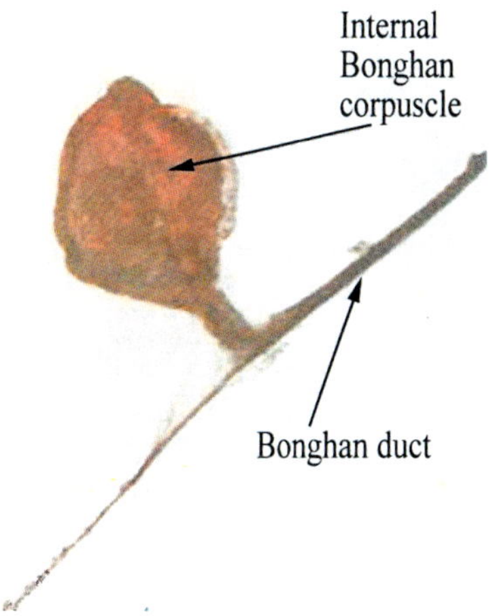

Figure 29. Internal Bonghan corpuscle (x63)

2) The corpuscle contains basophile granules of various sizes, and small and spherical nucleus-like structures (Figure 30). Cell elements are also recognized. These are myelopoietic and lymphogenetic cells in different stages of differentiation, that is, granulopoietic, monopoietic, erythrogenic and lymphopoietic elements and megakaryocytes (Figure 31).

It has been revealed that these cells of hematopoietic series alone are not found in the internal Bonghan corpuscle. The cell elements vary according to the kind of corpuscles.

In some part of the corpuscle, a cluster of cells similar to peculiar parenchymal cells can be seen. For instance, in the internal Bonghan [p22] corpuscles of the liver are found cell elements similar in structure to the liver cell. Sometimes they co-exist with cells of hemopoeitic series.

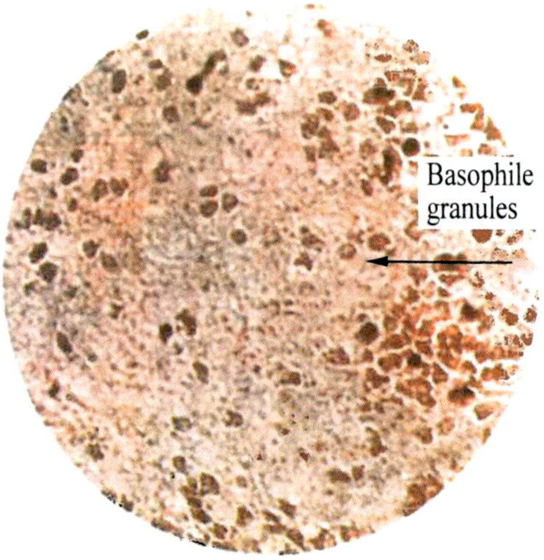

Figure 30. Internal Bonghan corpuscle (x400)

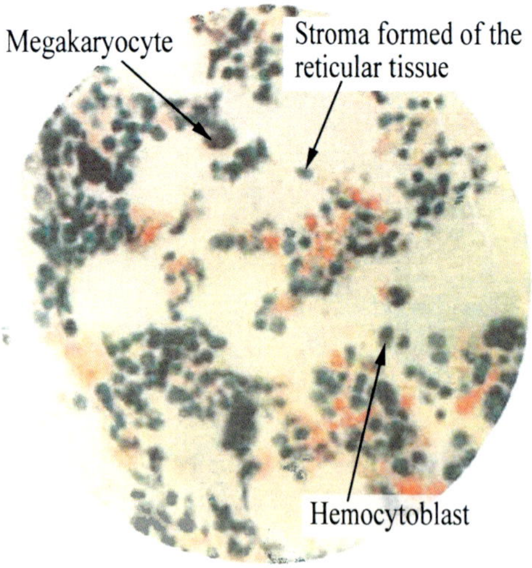

Figure 31. Internal Bonghan corpuscle (Giemsa stain) (x400)

The internal Bonghan corpuscle with the cluster of hemopoietic and other special cells is also found among the internal corpuscles of the abdominal aorta (Figure 32).

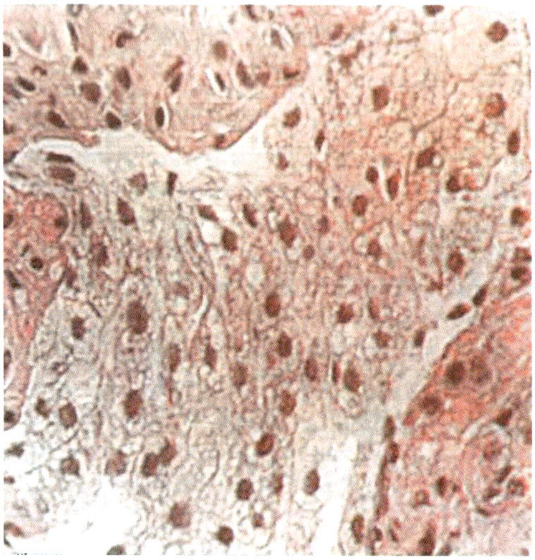

Figure 32. Internal Bonghan corpuscle (x400)

Particularly striking is the fact that these corpuscles contain fine chromaffine granules.

3) The stroma of the internal Bonghan corpuscle, like that of other hemopoietic organs, consists of undifferentiated reticular tissue. The outer membrane of the corpuscle is very thin.

4) The structure of the internal Bonghan corpuscle differs according to its maturity.

Examined under an electron microscope, the stroma of the internal corpuscle appears to be a network of fine fibres of high electron density mixed with small granules of various shapes and large ones of high electron density.

V. Intra-external Bonghan corpuscle

1. Anatomical observations of intra-external Bonghan corpuscle

Those profund Bonghan corpuscles, which are free from the surrounding tissues and exist independently of the path of the vessels, are called the intra-external Bonghan corpuscles.

The intra-external Bonghan corpuscles are linked up with the intra-external Bonghan ducts. Some of them are connected with the ducts at both ends, and in certain cases, several ducts are simultaneously linked with them. In the former case the corpuscle is about 0.3-1.0 mm X 0.1-0.5 mm in size and in the latter, 0.6-2.5 mm X 0.3-1.5 mm.

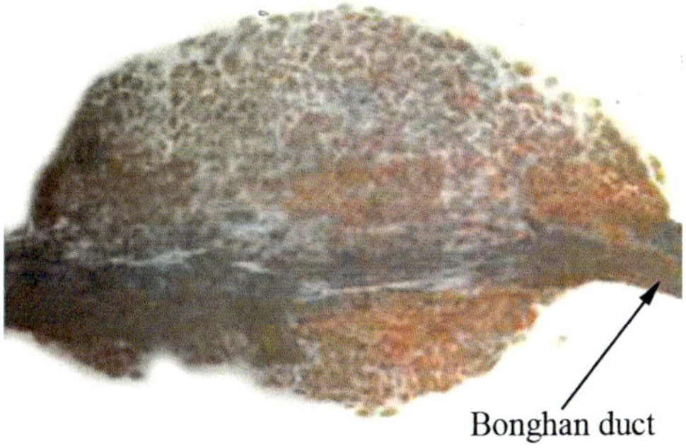

Figure 33. Intra-external Bonghan corpuscle (x160)

The former case is seen more frequently than the latter. In the latter case the intra-external Bonghan corpuscles are connected with three to seven ducts as a rule, and they take fusiform or polygonal irregular form and are semi-transparent, lactescent or lightly reddish in their colour.

The corpuscles connected at both ends by ducts are either fusiform or oval (Figure 33).

There are cases, when only one end of a corpuscle is connected to [p23] the duct. One finds very often several intra-external Bonghan ducts, which are intersected and covered with thin connective tissue.

2. Histological structure of intra-external Bonghan corpuscle

The intra-external Bonghan corpuscle is also formed basically by the ramifications and anastomoses of Bonghan ductules.

A. The Bonghan duct sinus contains basophile structures, either small or somewhat large spherical nucleus-like structures and other cells. And cells of different sizes with pale cytoplasm are scattered or crowded.

B. The stroma of the corpuscle consists of a fine fibrous network and besides nuclei of the connective tissue cells, audiophile cells can also be seen there.

The specimens of corpuscles are classified into several forms as follows:

(1) The contents of the Bonghan duct are not recognized but merely ducts and duct sinuses are seen.

(2) Spherical nucleus-like structures are crowded in the ducts.

(3) In the Bonghan duct sinus there exist cells with pale cytoplasm and when they are localized in the central part of the corpuscle, the structure of the stroma looks more plainly.

It is understood that different amounts and kinds of cell elements are to be seen in the corpuscle according to the degree of maturity of the corpuscle.

The striking fact in the intra-external corpuscle is that fine Bonghan ductules are interlaced reticulately inside the corpuscle and they are filled with basophile granules (Figure 34).

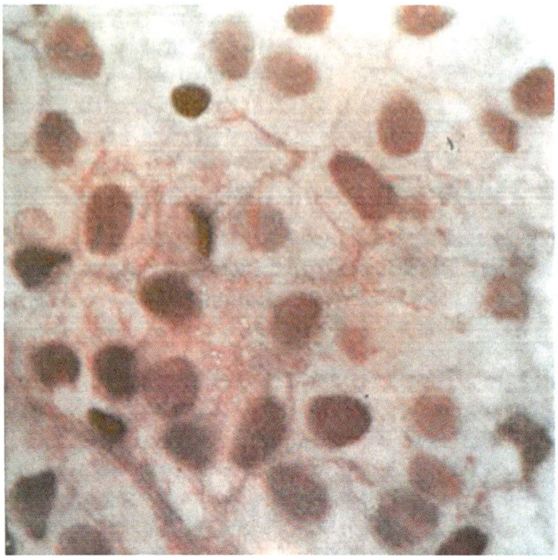

Figure 34. Intra-external Bonghan corpuscle (x1,000)

VI. Neural Bonghan corpuscle

The neural Bonghan corpuscle looks light Yellowish-white and semitransparent, the larger one measuring 0.5-1.0 mm in major axis and 0.2-0.5 mm in minor axis, and is of either an oval or spindle form. This corpuscle is connected with two to four neural Bonghan ducts in a bipolar or multipolar way. Inside the corpuscle, chiefly cells with pale cytoplasm, basophile granules and small nucleus-like structures are [p24] seen. Surrounding the corpuscle is the thin outer membrane of the connective tissues containing elongated ellipsoidal or fusiform nuclei of cells. This membrane is transformed to the periductium of the neural Bonghan duct (Figure 35).

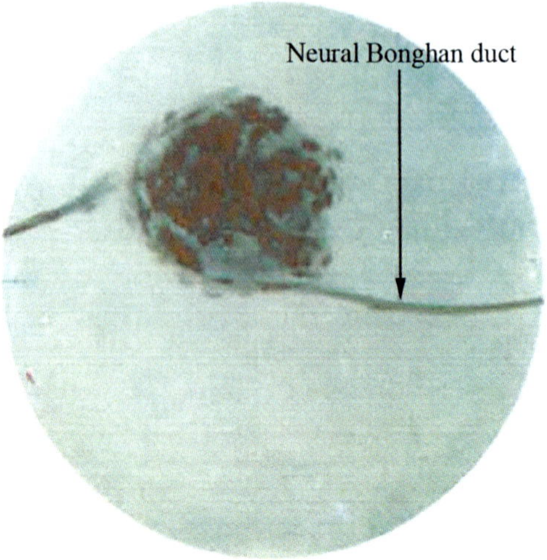

Figure 35. Neural Bonghan corpuscle (x160)

VII. Intraorganic Bonghan corpuscle

1. Anatomical observations of intraorganic Bonghan corpuscle

The intraorganic Bonghan corpuscle means the corpuscle located in the internal and other organs.

The corpuscle measures 0.1-0.5 mm in size. It is not sharply distinguished from the surrounding tissue in the living body but only under the stereomicroscope can it be distinguished by its external features such as colour, consistency and compactness.

The intraorganic Bonghan corpuscle appears more compact than the surrounding tissue and some of the corpuscles under the outer membrane of internal organs can be seen from outside. Somewhat large are the intraorganic Bonghan corpuscles found in the connective tissue around the comparatively large blood vessels in an internal organ; small-sized Bonghan corpuscles are to be seen on the Bonghan ducts coming out of these corpuscles.

2. Histological structure of intraorganic Bonghan corpuscle

The outstanding feature of the intraorganic Bonghan corpuscle is that it is the smallest in size and the simplest in structure among the Bonghan corpuscles.

There are granular and filiform basophile structures in the corpuscle. Similar structures are also found in the intraorganic corpuscles of the heart, liver, spleen, kidney, stomach, large and small intestines, testicles, ovary, and the suprarenal body.

In the intraorganic Bonghan corpuscle is occasionally to be seen cells similar to the young cells of the relevant organ. [p25]

VIII. Morphological dynamics of Bonghan corpuscle

When carefully studied, the various histological structures of the Bonghan corpuscles could be regarded as different stages of one dynamic process.

To prove this, studies were done mainly on the internal and superficial Bonghan corpuscles. The structures of the internal Bonghan corpuscles which were taken out of the same region of blood vessels were compared with each other, and the discernible corpuscles in lymphatic vessels were observed through the wall for a long period of time.

1. Morphological dynamics of Bonghan corpuscle in lymphatic vessels

First Stage:

The Bonghan corpuscle appears to be an opaque and milk-white clot and its boundary is not distinguished. Histological study of the corpuscle at this moment reveals a stage at which no cell element is to be seen except basophile granules in growth (Figure 36).

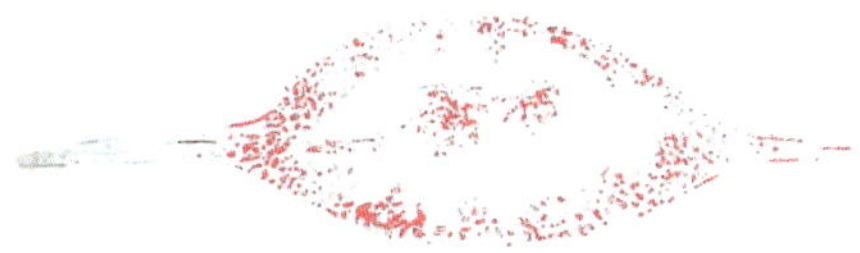

Figure 36. Morphological dynamics of the internal Bonghan duct (first stage)

Second Stage:

The Bonghan corpuscle is milk-white or yellowish at times and opaque. Its outer layer is hardly recognizable.

Basophile granules are scanty; basophile structures are crowded, and a part of them grows into small, nucleus-like structures (Figure 37).

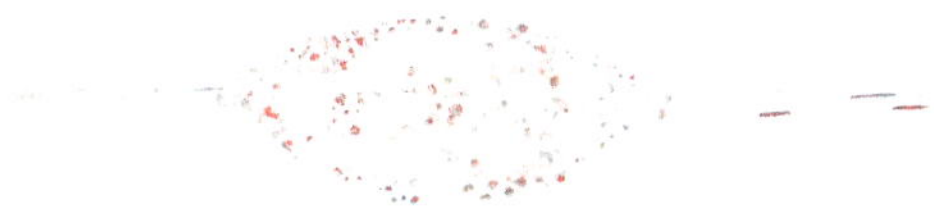

Figure 37. Morphological dynamics of the internal Bonghan duct (second stage)

Third Stage:

The corpuscle resembles a cluster of fat globules. It is soft in consistency, has smooth surface and glittering appearance.

Its connection with the Bonghan duct is clear and the formation of the outer membrane is recognizable. Basophile granules turn into small nucleus-like structures. The transition of small, nucleus-like structures to the form of nucleus is also recognized (Figure 38).

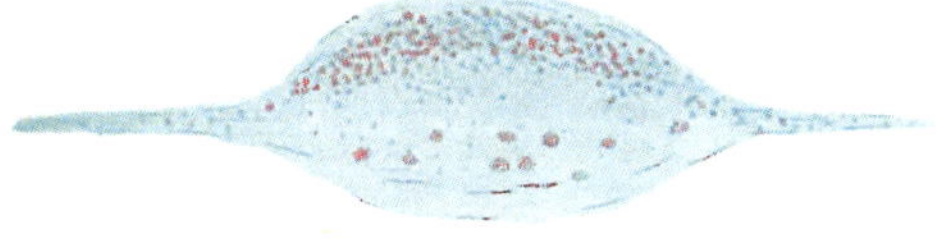

Figure 38. Morphological dynamics of the internal Bonghan duct (third stage)

Fourth Stage:

The corpuscle is either semi-transparent or transparent, and grayish-yellow, its contour being well distinguished.

Many lymphoid cells are found inside the corpuscle which is of an oval-shape (Figure 39). As time goes on, the corpuscle becomes opaque and grayish-white and the shape of the outer membrane begins to [p26] change. By this time, large, medium and tiny lymphocytes are observed to have been fully grown (Figure 40).

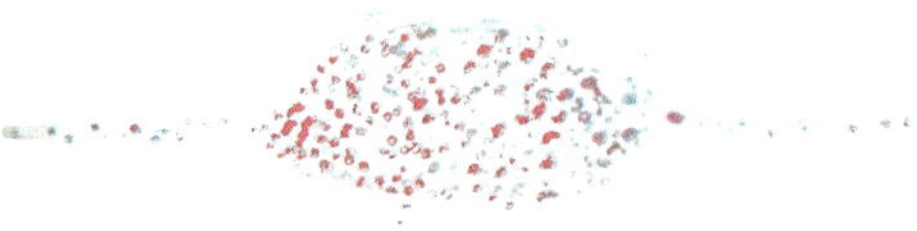

Figure 39. Morphological dynamics of the internal Bonghan duct (fourth stage -1)

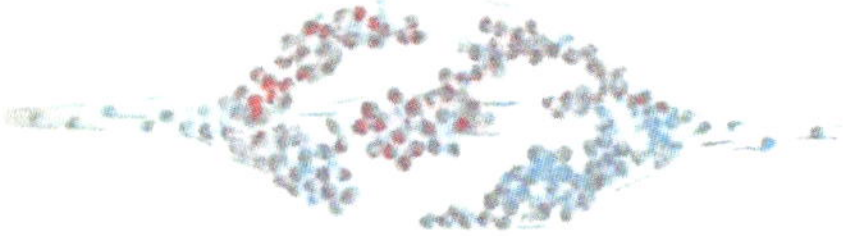

Figure 40. Morphological dynamics of the internal Bonghan duct (fourth stage -2)

Mature cells thrust outwards through the holes of the destroyed outer membrane. It is considered that such morphological dynamic process takes place in all Bonghan corpuscles of the living body.

2. Morphological dynamics of superficial Bonghan corpuscle

Having learned through observations that the superficial Bonghan corpuscles of a rabbit might assume a variety of structures, a continued observation of a definite corpuscle was done for a long period of time. In consequence it was ascertained that the structure of a corpuscle alters.

1) When observed in the living body, the boundary of a corpuscle is not clear but the corpuscle can be seen through epidermis.

A corpuscle is surrounded by numerous blood vessels and a stimulation to the corpuscle brings about active reaction of them.

2) The boundary of the corpuscle becomes somewhat clearer, cubic impression more accentuated. Rather dilated, but less blood vessels attend the corpuscle than in the foregoing case.

3) In the living body the epidermis covering the corpuscle appears more glittering and the surface is smooth. When touched, the corpuscle is felt considerably solid.

The cubic impression of the corpuscle becomes more accentuated, the inner substance is easy to recognize through outer layers and the surrounding blood vessels are less in number but remarkably dilated. [p27]

Part II. Various systems of Kyungrak

The afore-said constituent parts build various systems of Kyungrak: the internal Bonghan duct system, intra-external Bonghan duct system, external Bonghan duct system, neural Bonghan duct system and intra-organic Kyungrak system.

I. Internal Bonghan duct system

The internal Bonghan duct system accompanies the whole paths of blood and lymphatic vessels and is distributed in the organs.

This system is composed of the internal Bonghan ducts and the internal Bonghan corpuscles linked with each other by the ducts.

A blood vessel has usually one or two Bonghan ducts in it, whereas a thicker one several ducts. In general, an internal Bonghan duct comprises 1-15 Bonghan ductules, while a duct in a blood vessel of a certain region is made up of a bundle of scores of Bonghan ductules.

Where a blood vessel or a lymphatic vessel ramifies, so does the Bonghan duct.

There are two ways of bifurcation:

One is the dendroid ramification like the blood vessel and the other is the division of the ductule bundle as in nerves.

The flow of Bonghan liquor in the Bonghan duct generally coincides with the direction of blood flow, but the reverse phenomenon is also observed, e.g., the Bonghan liquor in the Bonghan duct of the suprarenal artery flows against the current of blood and goes out of the suprarenal body into the kidney through the internal Bonghan duct of the renal artery.

And it is noticed that the Bonghan liquor in the Bonghan duct of [p28] the large blood vessels reaching viscera flows against the current of blood.

These facts show that the internal Bonghan duct system, though located inside the vessels, has an order quite different from that of the vascular system.

More striking is the fact that Bonghan ducts go in and out of the blood vessels, penetrating their walls. This is demonstrated frequently in the abdominal aorta, in the peripheral blood vessels as well as in the lymphatic vessels. This leads to the conclusion that the formation of the internal Bonghan duct system is different from that of the vascular system. In the centre of the vascular system is situated the heart, but the same cannot be said of the internal Bonghan duct system. This system has no such centre as the heart. All the Bonghan ducts are not connected to form a single route but a number of different and specific routes. That is to say, the Bonghan liquor has many circulating routes and each route is linked with a different organ, whereas the circulating courses of blood connect all the organs and tissues to one common route. Some organs can have connections with many circulating routes, while others with less routes. For example, the endocrine organs are linked with many circulating routes. The Bonghan liquor from the ovary goes to the tissues of many organs (Figure 41, p.30 and Figure 42, p.31).

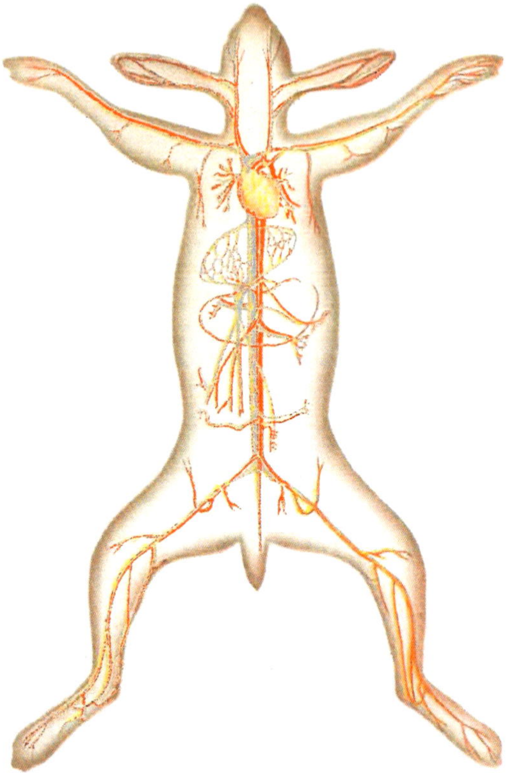

Figure 41. Internal Bonghan duct system

What attracts particular attention in the internal Bonghan corpuscle is immature blood cells.

Besides myeloid elements, lymphoid elements are also observed. This suggests that an active hematopoietic process takes place here. But cell division is hardly to be observed, whereas a good deal of basophile granules and small nucleus-like structures are to be seen.

When the erythrocytes in the bone marrow and peripheral blood are destroyed with phenylhydrazine, erythropoiesis is activated in the internal Bonghan corpuscles and these corpuscles are enlarged.

On the contrary, anaemia develops gradually when the internal Bonghan duct system is injured.

These data prove that hematopoiesis is one of the important functions of the internal Bonghan duct system.

II. Intra-external Bonghan duct system

The intra-external Bonghan duct system, independent of the paths of vessels and nerves, is distributed all over the body like a network.

The intra-external Bonghan duct is little different in structure [p29] from the internal Bonghan duct, and it is actually connected with the latter, getting through the wall of the blood vessel.

Its distribution shows a definite order though it is found in all parts of the body including the cervical, thoracal and abdominal regions, and thus forming very complex reticula.

The intra-external Bonghan ducts, in their courses, are linked with the intra-external Bonghan corpuscles, and are directly connected with all the internal organs within the body cavities, endocrine glands, the muscles of the abdominal wall, peritoneum, diaphragm and pleura.

The intra-external Bonghan ducts in the cervical region are connected with the intra-external Bonghan ducts in the chest, while descending along the bundles of nerves and blood vessels around the trachea and oesophagus.

These ducts in the chest, which are less in number than in the abdomen, descend towards the abdomen, passing by the auricles of the heart at the height of the incisura jugularis of the sternal bone, and running along both sides of the inferior vena cava. In this course, some branches of the intra-external Bonghan ducts go into the pericardium, myocardium, lung, trachea, oesophagus, large blood vessels and pleura.

Reaching the diaphragm, some of them penetrate it and the rest is linked with the intra-external Bonghan ducts in the abdomen through the aortic and oesophageal openings.

The intra-external Bonghan ducts are distributed more densely in the abdomen than in the chest, and they assume various forms on the front and back sides of the liver and the stomach.

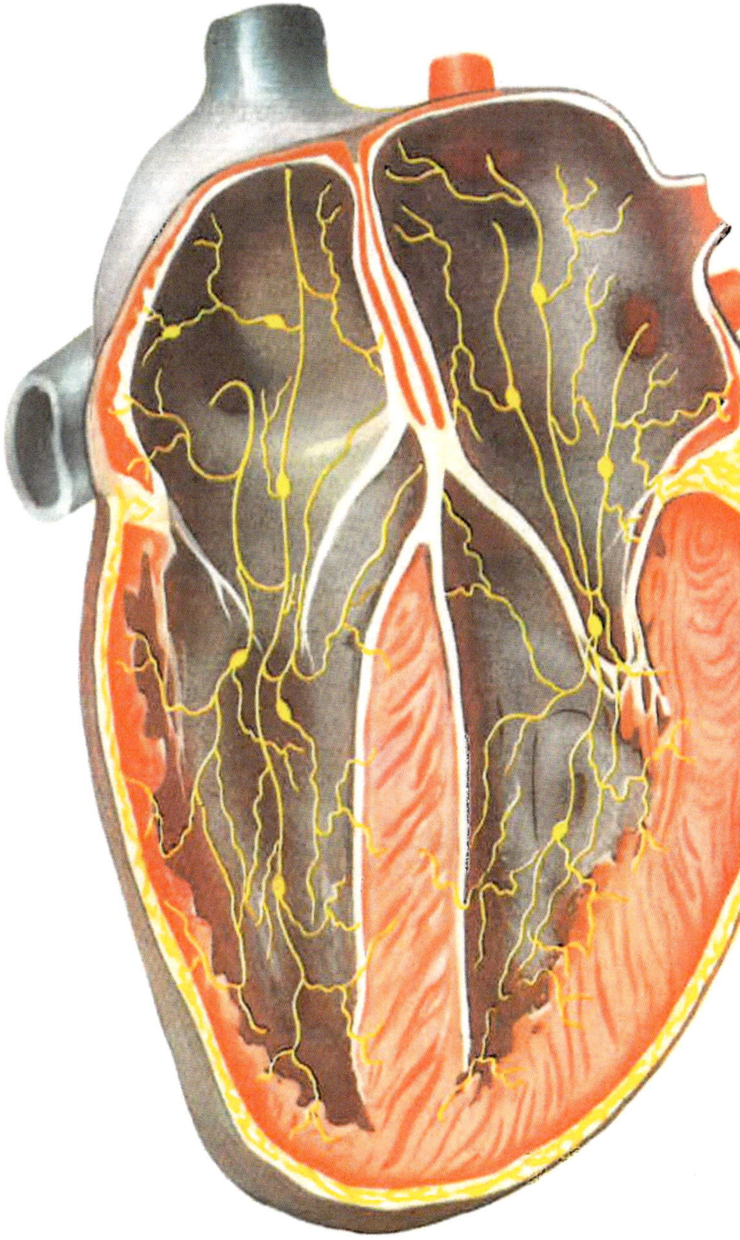

Figure 42. Internal Bonghan duct system (cardiac cavity)

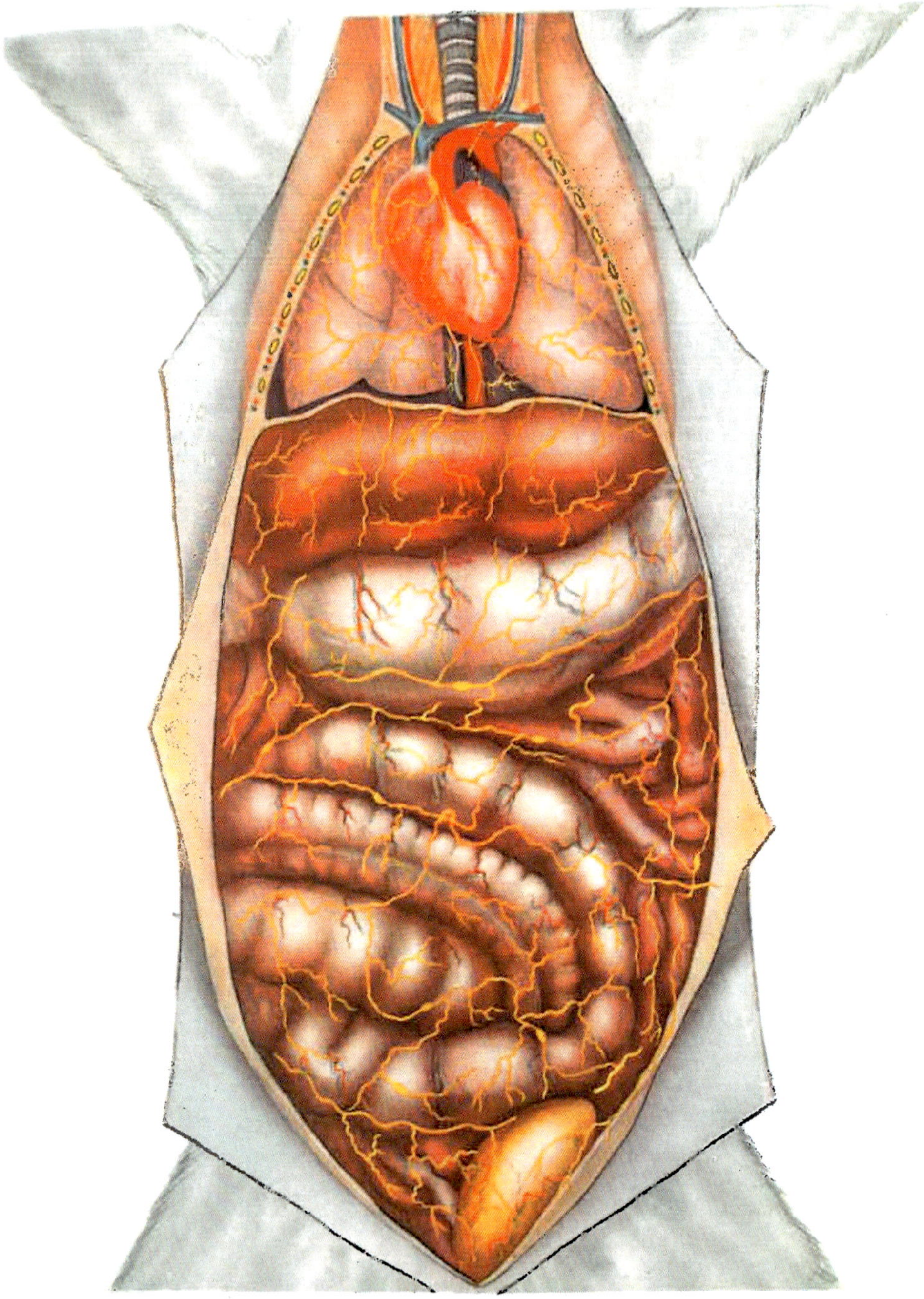

Figure 43. Intra-external Bonghan duct system

The intra-external Bonghan ducts widely distributed on the surface of the stomach and intestines send out numerous branches to form a dense network, which extends to various organs, linking them with one another. Part of the network of Bonghan ducts ramifies into the connective tissues around the large blood vessels.

The intra-external Bonghan ducts lie in a free state, but they stick to the surface of organs and the wall of the blood vessels only in the region where they branch off (Figure 43 and Figure 44).

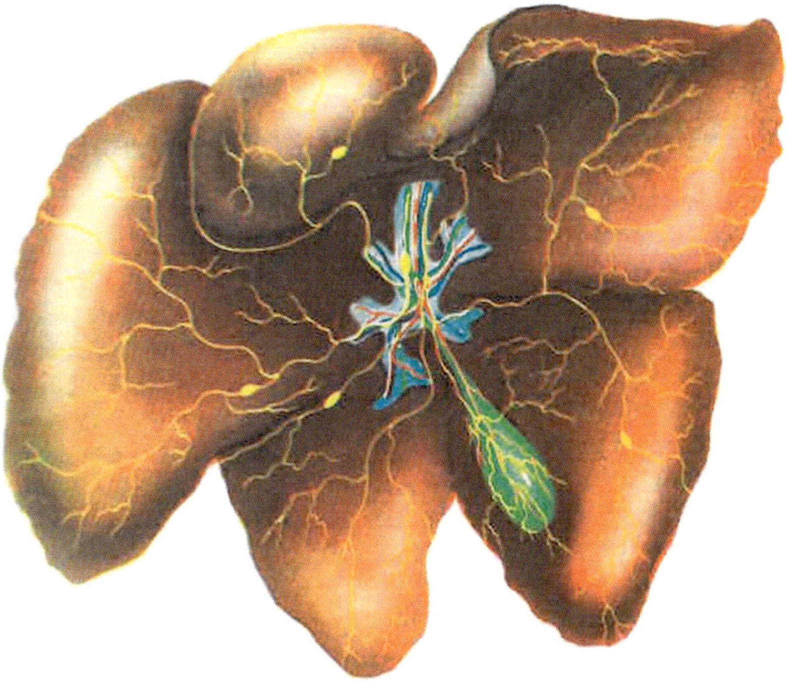

Figure 44. Intra-external Bonghan duct system of the liver

III. External Bonghan duct system

The external Bonghan ducts are distributed throughout the body, running along, or running independently of, the blood vessels and nerves. They link the external Bonghan corpuscles. Around the large [p30] blood vessels of the abdomen, for instance, the external Bonghan ducts link Bonghan corpuscles, running in four to six lines.

Running along blood vessels, the external Bonghan ducts send out branches to all internal organs including the heart, liver, gall bladder, and suprarenal body.

Those ducts which are located in the corium link directly superficial Bonghan corpuscles together, regardless of blood vessels and nerves, and some of them, penetrating the muscle, link themselves with profund Bonghan ducts.

IV. Neural Bonghan duct system

As in other organs, internal and external Bonghan ducts are distributed in the nervous system.

Besides these, a peculiar neural Bonghan duct system is found in the nervous system. In the central nervous system, the neural Bonghan ducts are distributed in the brain and spinal cord running in a free state through the central canal, cerebral ventricles, and subarachnoid space along the circulating route of the cerebrospinal liquor. And some of the ducts are linked with the Bonghan ducts under perineurium and with those between nerve fibres in the peripheral nervous system.

They are called neural Bonghan ducts, and the corpuscles linked by them, the neural Bonghan corpuscles.

The neural Bonghan ducts in the brain are connected with those in the spinal cord. In other words, the neural Bonghan duct in IV cerebral ventricle is linked downwards with that in the central canal of the spinal cord and upwards with that in III cerebral ventricle through the cerebral aqueduct. While running along the median sulcus at the floor of IV ventricle, the duct is connected with the neural Bonghan corpuscles below the anterior medullary velum, from which it obliquely crosses the stria medullaris and goes over the eminentia medialis, and then it is distributed in both cerebellar hemispheres.

Some of their branches, running through the chorioid tissue of IV ventricle, enter subarachnoid space through the sulcus medianus and sulcus limitans of the rhombencephalon.

In III ventricle the duct is connected, through the inter-ventricular foramen, with the neural Bonghan duct in the lateral ventricle, and through the cerebral aqueduct, with that in IV ventricle.

While running parallel with the tela chorioidea of III ventricle, the [p31] neural Bonghan duct gives forth a branch which makes its way to the subarachnoid space along the dorsal side of the pineal body, penetrating the lamina epithelialis of the chorioid plexus. In the lower region, while running along the recessus infundibuli and recessus opticus, this duct diverges into the posterior perforated substance, the anterior part of the crus cerebri, the mammillary body, and the tuber cinereum, etc., and is mainly distributed in the diencephalon.

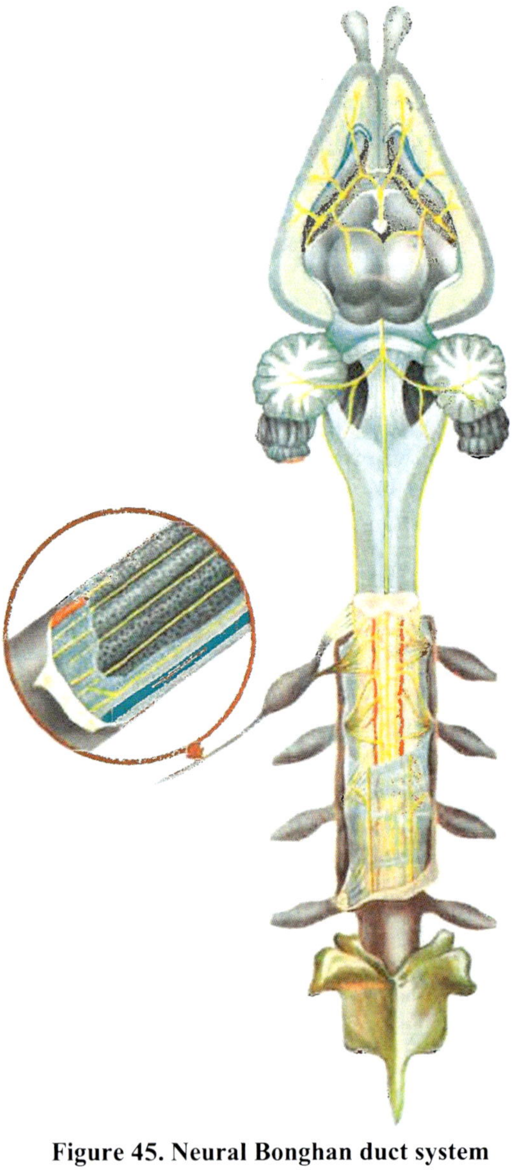

Figure 45. Neural Bonghan duct system

In the lateral ventricle the neural Bonghan duct joins that in III ventricle through the inter-ventricular foramen, and branches out in the anterior horn, central part, posterior and inferior horns of the lateral ventricle to diverge in the frontal, parietal, occipital and temporal lobes of the cerebrum respectively. Some branches of the neural Bonghan duct enter the chorioid plexus of the lateral ventricle. The neural Bonghan duct entering the subarachnoid space is linked with the neural Bonghan corpuscles to form a network and is distributed in the brain tissue penetrating the pia mater.

The neural Bonghan ducts of the spinal cord run along the central canal, linking themselves with those of the brain in the upper region and are distributed in the spinal cord, connecting the corpuscles in different parts.

Some branches penetrate into subarachnoid space through the spinal cord and some, after running along the spinal nerves, turn to the neural Bonghan ducts of peripheral nerve, running between the nerve fibres.

The neural Bonghan ducts in the subarachnoid space of the spinal cord form a dense network and some of them ramify to be connected with the neural Bonghan ducts of the peripheral nerves.

The neural Bonghan duct in the central canal does not send out branches in accordance with the segmental ramifications of the spinal nerves, but it usually gives off a branch in every two or three segments.

The neural Bonghan duct system is communicated with other Bonghan duct systems as well. For instance, when dye is injected into the internal Bonghan duct of the ovary, it reaches the neural Bonghan duct, and when dye is introduced into the neural Bonghan duct system, it moves to the intra-external Bonghan duct system in the abdominal and thoracic cavities (Figure 45 and Figure 46).

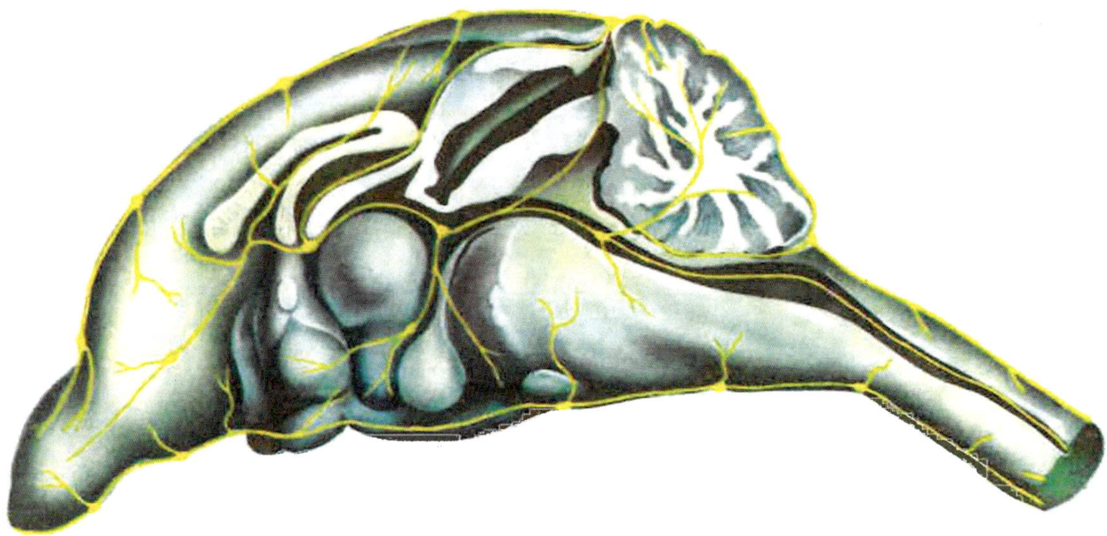

Figure 46. Neural Bonghan duct system

Neural Bonghan ducts within peripheral nerves

The neural Bonghan duct system which has been in the central nervous system is connected with the peripheral nervous system which is distributed throughout the organs. [p32]

The neural Bonghan ducts run with the loose connective tissues of epineurium and perineurium and also lie in the connective tissue of endoneurium (Figure 47 and Figure 48).

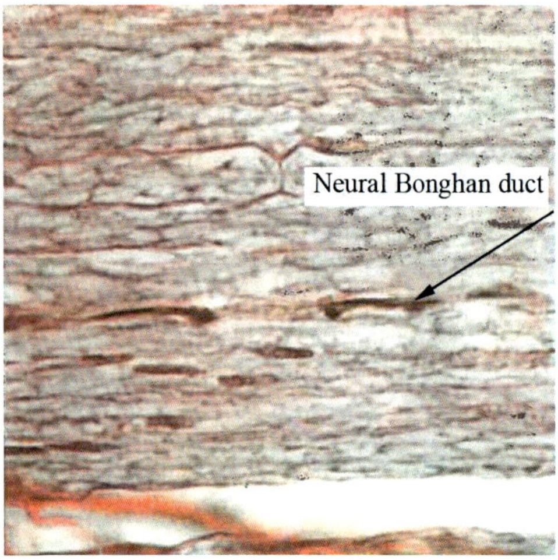

Figure 47. Neural Bonghan duct (in the peripheral nerves) (x400)

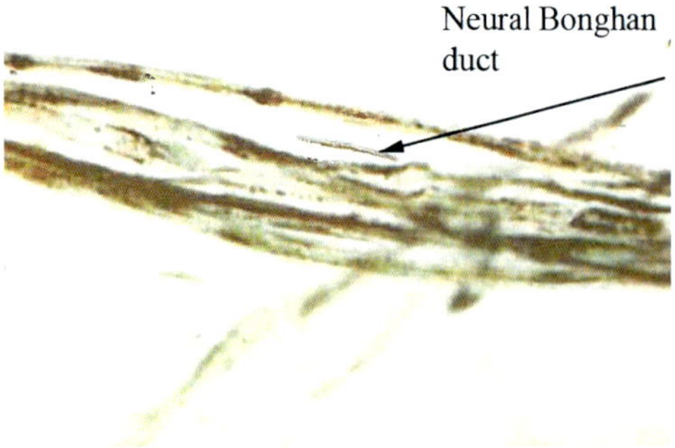

Figure 48. Neural Bonghan duct (in the peripheral nerves) (x400)

The Bonghan ductules of the endoneurium follow almost the same paths of nerve fibres, but sometimes, they cross nerve fibres transversely or curve sideways.

It is difficult to distinguish the Bonghan ductule unless the nerve fibre is separated, because the ductule sticks to the endoneural sheath. And it usually runs singly.

The ductule is very fine and its endothelial nuclei are rarely found. The ductule measures about 2 microns in calibre and its endothelial nucleus is rod-shaped, and 15-20 microns in length.

In the histological sections stained with hematoxylin after silver impregnation the Bonghan ductule is not well impregnated but appears transparent and light blue.

The endothelial nuclei of the ductule are stained deeply with hematoxylin, making it difficult to observe the nucleoli.

The characteristics of the Bonghan ductule are distinguished clearly from those of the nerve fibres, connective tissue fibres, blood and lymphatic vessels.

V. Interrelations among various systems

Various systems of Kyungrak mentioned above are related with each other to form an integrated system. For instance, the internal Bonghan ducts penetrate the walls of arterioles and venules and meet the external Bonghan ducts at the intraorganic Bonghan corpuscles.

And in the large blood vessels also the internal Bonghan ducts come outwards to be linked with the intra-external Bonghan ducts.

The external and the internal Bonghan duct are connected with each other in the superficial Bonghan corpuscle as well.

It has been confirmed that the neural Bonghan ducts are linked with the intra-external Bonghan ducts.

Thus all the systems of Kyungrak are interlinked.

VI. Kyungrak system within organs

Though the distribution of the Kyungrak system within each organ is specific, it has a series of common features. [p33]

Various systems of Kyungrak are distributed together in the same organ. Namely, the internal Bonghan duct penetrates into an organ through the blood vessel, while the external Bonghan duct enters the same organ, after running along, or running independently of, the blood vessel.

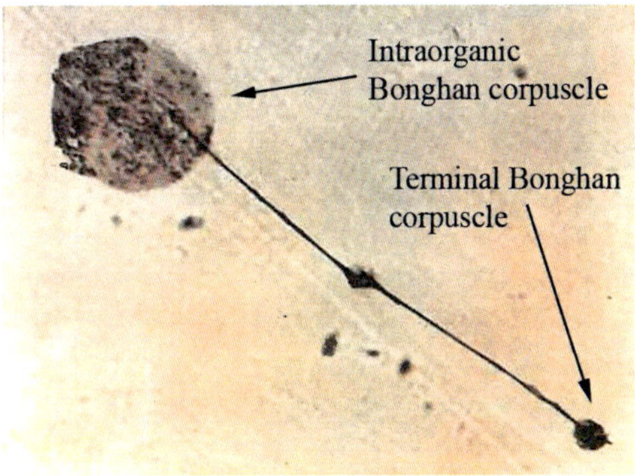

Figure 49. Terminal Bonghan corpuscle (in the suprarenal body) (x160)

The intra-external Bonghan duct enters the organ, sending out many branches. In the organ the internal Bonghan duct, penetrating the wall of the arteriole, links up with an intraorganic Bonghan corpuscle, from which it again penetrates into the venule. To the intraorganic corpuscle is connected the external Bonghan duct entering the organ.

It seems that the branches of the intra-external Bonghan duct anastomose with the external Bonghan duct.

The Bonghan duct leaving the intraorganic Bonghan corpuscle ramifies and reaches a number of minute intraorganic corpuscles (called the terminal Bonghan corpuscle) (Figure 49).

The fine Bonghan ductules running out of the terminal Bonghan corpuscles (terminal Bonghan ductules) are directly linked to the cell nuclei (Figure 50).

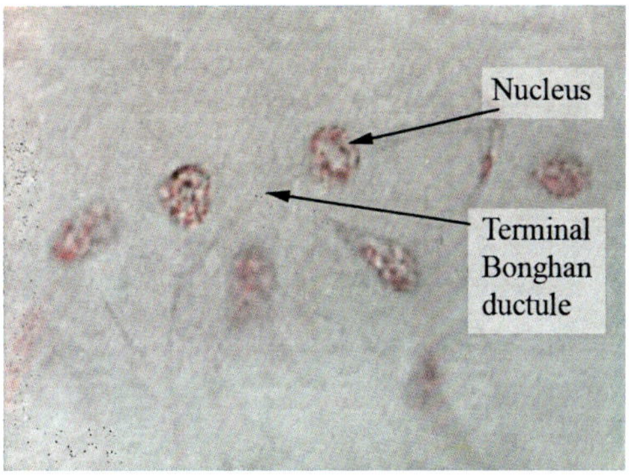

Figure 50. Terminal Bonghan ductule (in the suprarenal body) (x1,000)

A fine Bonghan ductule (terminal Bonghan ductule) comes out of the cell nucleus and it again passes through a tiny Bonghan corpuscle (terminal Bonghan corpuscle).

Numerous terminal Bonghan corpuscles are located in the organs, each of them being linked only with the cells within a definite range.

Between the intraorganic and the terminal Bonghan corpuscle lies usually one, sometimes two or three, small Bonghan corpuscle.

Having entered an internal organ, the external Bonghan ducts bring into shape of big intraorganic Bonghan corpuscles under the capsule of the organ or around the relatively large blood vessels. These corpuscles are linked with the intraorganic Bonghan corpuscles mentioned above.

The terminal Bonghan ductule gets thinner and enters cytoplasm, penetrating the cell membrane, and penetrates into the karyoplasm through the nuclear membrane. These ductules seem to form a network in the nucleus.

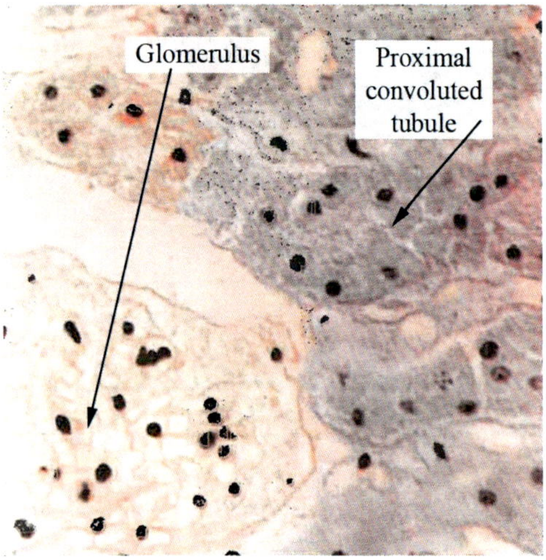

Figure 51. Changes in nuclei after cutting the Bonghan duct (in the kidney) (x400)

The terminal Bonghan ductule is filled with Feulgen positive granules and on its wall lie small endothelial nuclei.

When stain is injected into an intraorganic Bonghan corpuscle, it reaches cell nucleus and from there it again flows out of the cell through the fine Bonghan ductule linked with the nucleus.

In order to prove this, a Bonghan duct was cut and the result was examined. [p34]

When an internal Bonghan duct entering a parenchymal organ is severed, histologic changes are noticed in the associated organ.

When an internal Bonghan duct in portal vein is cut, the liver cell slightly enlarges in size and cytoplasm gets turbid in a day, karyolysis occurs in some cell nuclei, leading to the destruction of cells.

Three days after the cutting there takes place serious vacuolar degeneration in the parenchymal cells of the liver as a whole.

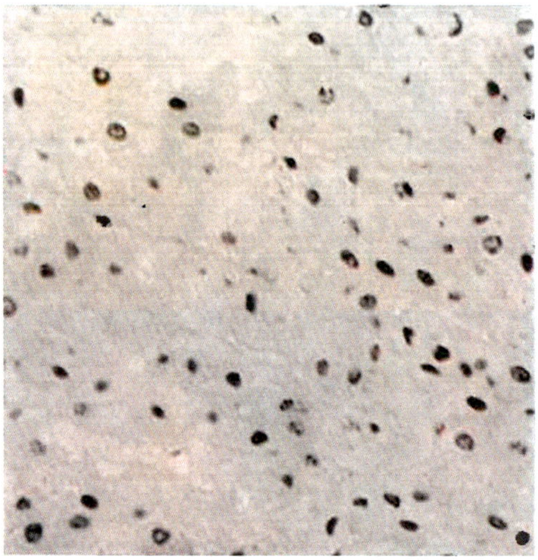

Figure 52. Changes in nuclei after cutting the Bonghan duct (in zona fasciculata of the suprarenal body) (x400)

When the external and the internal Bonghan duct distributed in the kidney are severed, necrosis of the convoluted uriniferous tubules and of the renal corpuscles is observed in the cortex of kidney, and the uriniferous tubules lose their nuclei thoroughly, while preserving their form.

The epithelial nuclei of the uriniferous tubules in medullary substance disappear entirely or are destroyed partly (Figure 51).

In case of the severance of the external and the internal Bonghan duct located in the suprarenal body, the terminal Bonghan ductules connected with nuclei in zona glomerulosa disappear in the early stage, and the nuclei become pyknotic and are destroyed or lost.

The basophile structures, large or small, slightly stained with basic dyes, appear in the region where the cells are destroyed.

The same can be said of zona fasciculata and zona reticularis (Figure 52). [p35]

Part III. Various systems of Kyungrak and their roles

Judging from the anatomico-histological characteristics, it is quite obvious that the influence of circulation of Bonghan liquor on the organs and tissues will have the greater significance for the Kyungrak system to play its role.

To clarify the whole aspect of this process, the biochemical composition of Bonghan liquor was analyzed, its path of circulation traced and the effect of a direct stimulus to a Bonghan duct on the functioning of the organ concerned was observed. And the influence of the cutting of a Bonghan duct on the organ concerned was studied and the conductibility of the Bonghan duct assisting the circulation of the liquor was also examined.

I. Biochemical composition of Bonghan liquor

A Bonghan duct of a rabbit was isolated and dissolved in citric acid-sucrose solution. The walls and nuclei of the duct were removed from this solution and the remaining liquor was studied.

1. Nitrogen, sugar and lipid contents of Bonghan liquor

Total nitrogen, nonprotein nitrogen, sugar and lipids were estimated by micro-Kjeldahl, Hagedorn-Jensen, and Bang method respectively.

The results are shown in Table 1. [p36]

As is seen in Table 1, the Bonghan liquor contains much protein and nonprotein nitrogen and a considerable amount of sugar and lipids.

Table 1. Contents (%)

Total nitrogen	3.12 - 3.40
Nonprotein nitrogen	0.10 - 0.17
Lipids	0.57 - 1.00
Reduced sugar	0.10 - 0.12

2. Total content of hyaluronic acid in Bonghan liquor

Ehrlich's direct-method as well as the ion exchange chromatography were applied in analyzing hyaluronic acid. The former is a well-known express-method but is not free from a number of defects in regard to accuracy. We, therefore, isolated and estimated hyaluronic acid chiefly by means of ion exchange chromatography.

For comparison, the clot of blood, the livers of rat and rabbit, the yolk and white of an egg, and the sperm of cattle were also examined. The results are shown in Table 2.

Compared to other tissues, the Bonghan liquor contains much hyaluronic acid, nearly as much as that contained in the cattle sperm.

It is of special interest that the Bonghan liquor in the intravascular Bonghan duct contains 25 times more hyaluronic acid than the clot of blood.

Table 2. Content of total hyaluronic acid (mg %)

Name of material	Ehrlich's direct-method		Ion exchange chromatography	
	Found	In literature	Found	In literature
Bonghan liquor	301.2 ± 20.1	—	170.4 ± 4.5	—
Clot of blood	39.7 ± 5.2	—	7.3 ± 0.8	—
Rat liver	116.3 ± 4.5	—	47.0 ± 2.5	30
Rabbit liver	41.0 ± 3.1	—	18.4 ± 3.5	—
The white	105.6 ± 7.0	100	41.6 ± 1.5	33
Yolk	320.0 ± 30.2	350	60.1 ± 1.7	61
Sperm of cattle	380.2 ± 27.7	420	178.3 ± 7.8	186

3. Free amino acid content in Bonghan liquor

Qualitative analysis of free amino acids was carried out by means of two-dimensional paper chromatography; solvent systems were [p37] n-butanol-glacial acetic acid-water and phenol-water.

The quantitative analysis of each free amino acid was done both by high voltage paper electrophoresis and one-dimensional paper chromatography. PH of the buffer solution for electrophoresis was 6.5, consisting of pyridine, glacial acetic acid and water.

Electrophoresis was carried out at the temperature of 0°C during 120 minutes (40 v/cm, 3 mA/cm).

One-dimensional ascending paper chromatography with the solvent system of n-butanol-glacial acetic acid-water was done during 24 hours and the procedure was repeated three times in each experiment. 0.2 per cent ninhydrin-acetone solution was sprayed and the spot of each amino acid was scanned through the spectrophotometer (λ: 360 mμ).

The results are shown in Table 3 and Figure 53, Figure 54 and Figure 55.

Table 3. Free amino acids in Bonghan liquor (mg %)

Amino acids	Content
leucine + isoleucine	14.56 ± 0.84
phenylalanine	4.92 ± 0.87
valine + methionine + tryptophane	15.07 ± 1.45
tyrosine	1.85 ± 0.09
alanine	12.00 ± 1.20
glutamic acid	7.39 ± 0.48
threonine	2.45 ± 0.45
glycine + serine	13.73 ± 2.32
asparagin	0.85 ± 0.04
lysine	4.14 ± 0.76
arginine	7.45 ± 0.91
aspartic acid	4.80 ± 0.33
glutamine	0.98 ± 0.07
histidine	1.85 ± 0.09
proline	—
cystine	3.57 ± 0.24

4. Composition of free mononucleotides in Bonghan liquor

The separation of free mononucleotides in the Bonghan liquor was done by both paper and ion exchange chromatographies. Solvent system for the paper chromatography was n-propanol-ammonia-water; spots of each mononucleotide were identified by the ultrachemiscope (Figure 56).

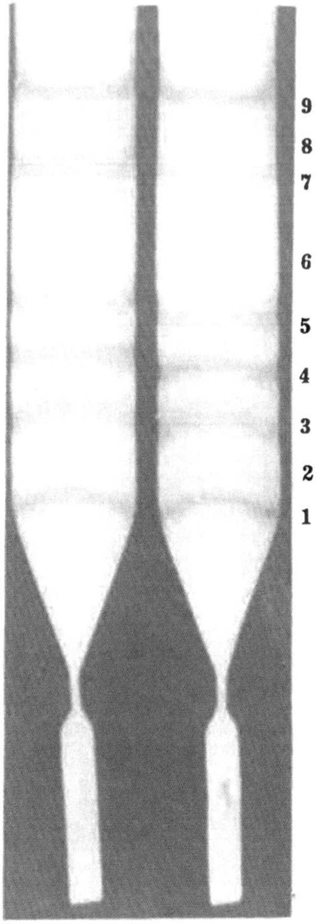

Figure 53. Paper chromatogram of free amino acids

Solvent system: n-butanol-glacial acetic acid-water

1. Cyctine
2. Asparagin
3. Glycine + Serin
4. Threonine
5. Alanine
6. Tyrosine
7. Valine + Methionine + Tryptophane
8. Pheylalanine
9. leucine + Isoleucine

Figure 54. High voltage paper electrophoregram of free amino acids

Buffer solution: Pyridine solution (pH 6.5)

1. Aspartic acid
2. Glutamic acid
3. Histidine
4. Lysine
5. Arginine

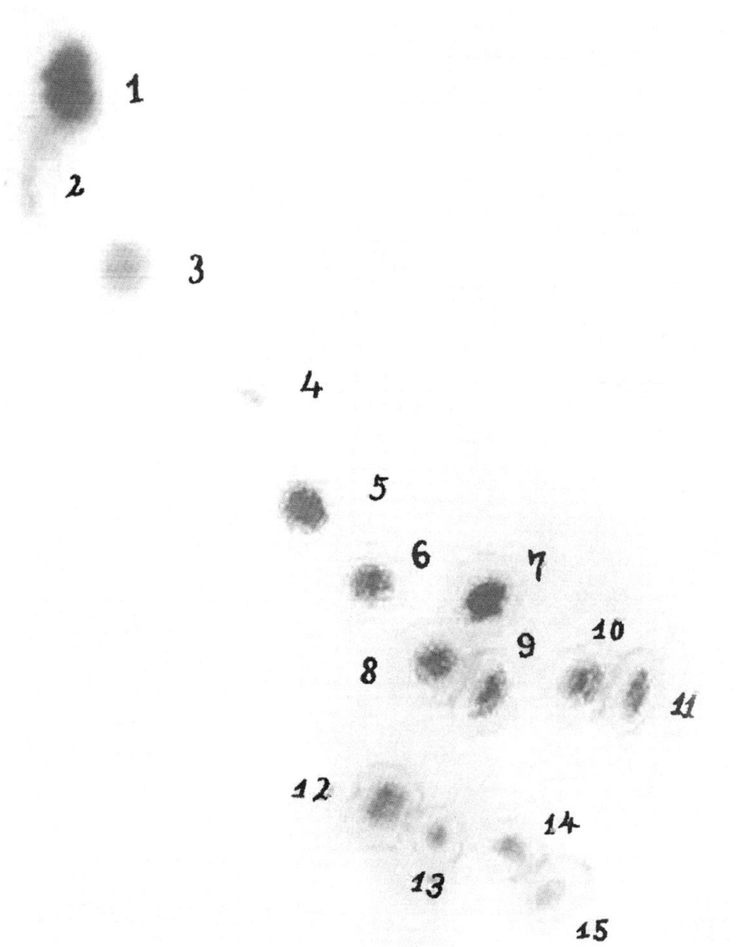

Figure 55. Two-dimensional chromatogram of free amino acids

Solvent system:
1) the first solvent — n-butanol-glacial acetic acid-water
2) the second solvent — saturated phenol solution

1. Leucine + Isoleucine
2. Phenylalanine
3. Valine + Methionine + Tryptophane
4. Tryosine
5. Alanine
6. Threnonine
7. Glutamin
8. Glycine
9. Serine
10. Aspartic acid
11. Asparagin
12. Arginine
13. Lysine
14. Histidine
15. Cystine

Figure 56 shows that through one-dimensional paper chromatography were separated adenosine diphosphate, guanosine polyphosphate, adenosine [p38] triphosphate and adenosine pentaphosphate from the Bonghan liquor. A number of other free nucleotides were separated by the ion exchanging method (ionites-Amberite IRA-400, Dowex-1).

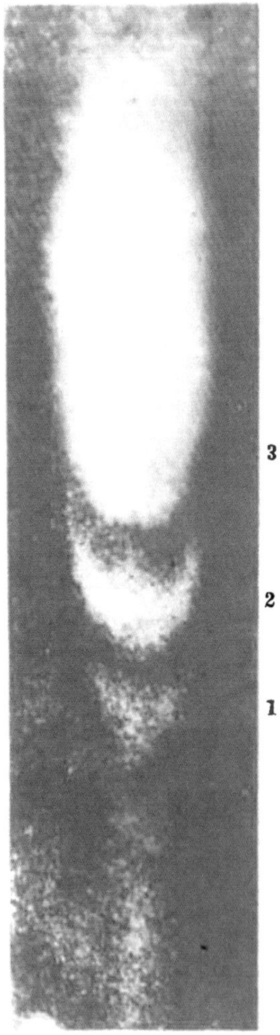

Figure 56. Paper chromatogram of free mononucleotides

Solvent system:
propanol-ammonia-water

1. Guanosine polyphosphate
2. Adenosine pentaphosphate
3. Adenosine triphosphate

0.5 N-formic acid, 1 N-formic acid, 4 N-formic acid, 4 N-formic acid + 0.2 N-ammonium formate and 4 N-formic acid + 0.6 N-ammonium formate were applied as solvent successively.

For the determination of individual free nucleotide, eluates of 0.6 ml per minute in auto-collector were combined together every five minutes and scanned through the ultraviolet spectrophotometer (λ: 260-280 mμ) (Figure 57).

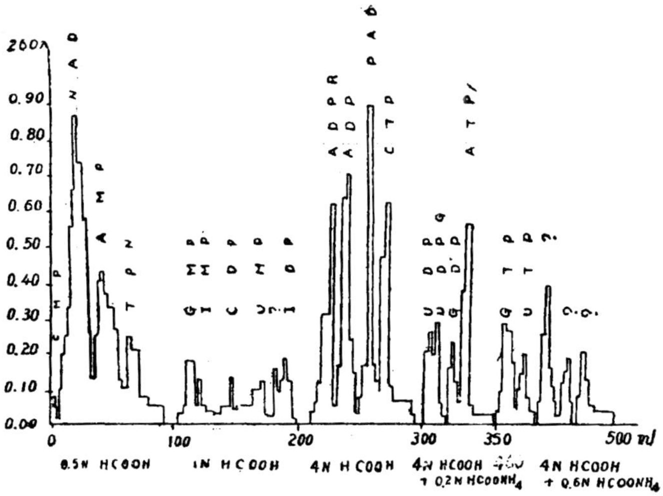

Figure 57. Free mononucleotide composition of the Bonghan liquor

Figure 57 indicates that the Bonghan liquor contains more than 16 kinds of free mononucleotides (cytosine monophosphate, nicotinadenine dinucleotide, adenosine monophosphate, inosine monophosphate, guanosine monophosphate, cytosine diphosphate, uridine monophosphate, adenosine diphosphate ribose, adenosine diphosphate, cytosine triphosphate, uridine diphosphate, uridine diphosphate hexosamine, guanosine diphosphate, adenosine triphosphate, guanosine triphosphate, uridine triphosphate). [p39]

5. Content of hormones in Bonghan liquor

The analyses of adrenalin and noradrenalin were performed by virtue of their selective absorption on aluminium hydroxide in alkaline medium. Bonghan liquor was separated from fresh Bonghan ducts under conditions of refrigeration and brought to analysis.

Together with the Bonghan liquor the superficial Bonghan corpuscles and other tissues were also analyzed for comparison (Table 4).

Table 4 indicates that adrenalin and noradrenalin are abundantly contained in the Bonghan liquor and in the superficial Bonghan corpuscle in comparison with the other tissues. It has been also established that the Bonghan liquor also contains corticosteroid, 17-ketosteroid and female hormone (estrogen).

Table 4. Content of adrenalin and noradrenalin (r/g)

Sample	Found		In literature	
	Adrenaline	Noradrenalin	Adrenalin	Noradrenalin
Bonghan liquor	0.22 - 0.40	0.60 - 1.50	—	—
Superficial Bonghan corpuscle	0.92 - 1.92	2.20 - 3.90	—	—
Heart	0.08 - 0.18	0.69 - 1.40	0.04 - 0.10	0.70 - 1.30
Blood	0.10 - 1.13	—	—	—

6. Base composition of DNA and nucleotide composition of RNA in Bonghan liquor

Separation of bases of DNA in the Bonghan liquor was done by paper chromatography with the solvent system of hydrochloric acid-methanol-water, and separation of mononucleotides of RNA was done by high voltage paper electrophoresis in the buffer solution of 0.5 mol acetic acid.

Localizations of the separated DNA bases and RNA nucleotides were ascertained either by the ultrachemiscope or photo development.

The data of analysis are shown in Figure 58 and Figure 59, and Table 5 and 6. [p40]

These data reveal that the molar ratio of purine to pyrimidine bases in DNA of the Bonghan liquor is approximately 1 and the ratio of adenine + thymine to guanine + cytosine is 1.35, i.e., the DNA of the Bonghan liquor is of AT-type.

The molar ratio in RNA of purine pyrimidine and that of guanylic acid + cytidylic acid to adenylic acid + uridylic acid are 1.05 and 1.47 respectively.

Besides nucleic acids, the Bonghan liquor contains proteins, carbohydrates, lipids and many free amino acids, and especially many mononucleotides not bound to cells.

These findings indicate that the Kyungrak system is intimately associated with the metabolism of nucleic acids.

Further, the Bonghan liquor contains hyaluronic acid and cortical and medullary hormones of the suprarenal body and female hormone (estrogen). These facts suggest that the Kyungrak system is also closely related to the endocrine system.

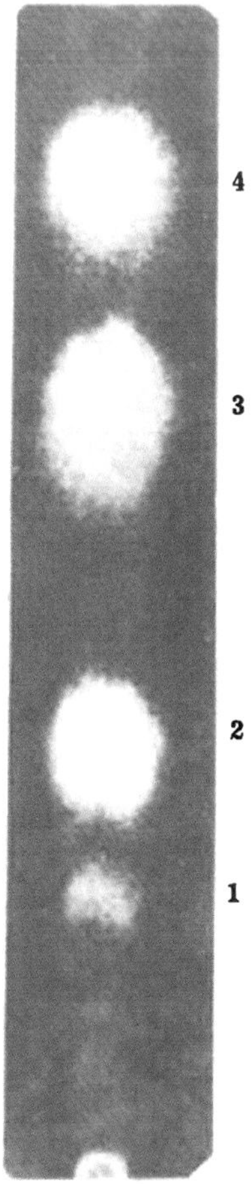

Figure 58. Paper chromatogram of the bases of deoxyribo-nucleic acid

Solvent system:
hydrochloric acid-methanol-water
1. Guanine
2. Adenine
3. Cytosine
4. Thymine

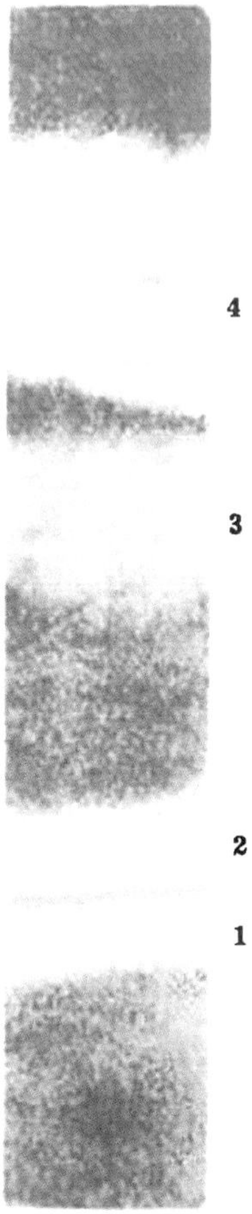

Figure 59. Paper electrophoregram of RNA mononucleotides

Buffer solution:
0.5 mol. acetic acid solution
1. Cytidylic acid
2. Adenylic acid
3. Guanylic acid
4. Uridylic acid

Table 5. Composition of DNA bases

Base	Molar ratio of bases (mol. %)
Guanine	21.80
Adenine	28.30
Cytosine	21.20
Thymine	28.70

Table 6. Composition of RNA nucleotides

Nucleotide	Molar ratio of nucleotides (mol. %)
Guanylic acid	30.21
Adenylic acid	21.10
Cytidylic acid	29.31
Uridylic acid	19.38

II. Conductibility of Bonghan duct

In order to make clear the conductibility of the Bonghan duct, we examined, first of all, the bioelectrical features of the Bonghan duct.

1. Bioelectrical features of Bonghan duct

An internal Bonghan duct was separated from a rabbit and placed on electrodes in a glass tube or in a damp chamber containing serum-saline solution, and then connected with a silver-chloride electrode. Then bio-electrical changes were recorded by means of a low-frequency [p41] amplifier and an electro-magnetic recorder.

It has been revealed that the specific bioelectrical changes in the Bonghan duct are not quite different from those observed in the superficial Bonghan corpuscle, i.e., "ㄱ", "ㄴ", and "ㄷ" waves were observed mixed.

But the bioelectrical changes in the Bonghan duct are generally of lower amplitude than those in the superficial Bonghan corpuscle, and the "ㄷ" wave was difficult to observe (Figure 60).

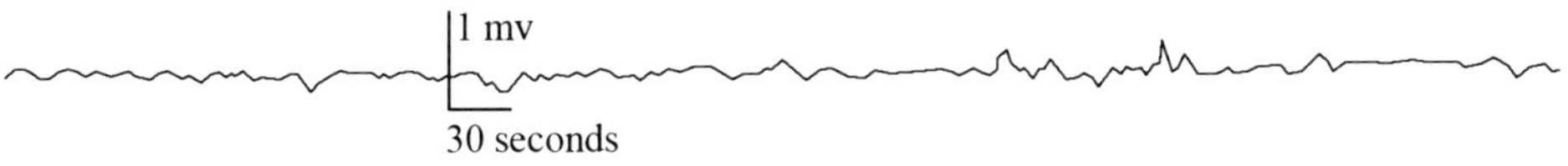

Figure 60. Bioelectrical changes recorded in the Bonghan duct

The "ㄴ" wave often appears in groups periodically when the Bonghan duct is stimulated.

Such bioelectrical changes in the isolated Bonghan duct get weaker with the lapse of time and usually subside within 30-40 minutes, unless the surrounding conditions are favourable enough to maintain the reaction. Bioelectrical changes bear various characters in accordance with the nature of stimuli.

At the temperature under 25°C the bio-electrical changes are apt to disappear. But the subsided bioelectrical phenomena revive when the temperature is raised right after their disappearance. When affected by various drugs the bioelectrical change becomes either accentuated or weakened.

Such effect of the stimuli depends upon the kind of chemicals applied as well as upon the conditions of the Bonghan duct prior to the stimulation. Chemical stimuli given to the Bonghan duct with pronounced bioelectrical changes often bring forth weaker or no change.

The same bioelectrical changes as in the case of the isolated specimen were also observed in the Bonghan ducts of the region where [p42] blood circulation was stopped through the slight ligature of the proximal and distal ends of the blood vessels.

Various patterns of bioelectrical changes are exhibited according to the position of the Bonghan duct.

All these results indicate that the bioelectrical changes also occur in the Bonghan duct just like in the superficial Bonghan corpuscle and the patterns of changes are nearly the same in both cases.

2. Bioelectrical analysis of conductibility of Bonghan duct

In order to clarify the conductibility of the Kyungrak system, experiments were done in stimulating isolated internal Bonghan ducts.

One end of an internal Bonghan duct, either isolated or exposed in the living body through blood vessel ligature, was connected to the apparatus for registration of bioelectrical changes, and the other end was stimulated either by electricity or by chemical drugs.

The electrical changes of minor amplitude follow closely these stimuli and those of major amplitude after a certain interval (Figure 61).

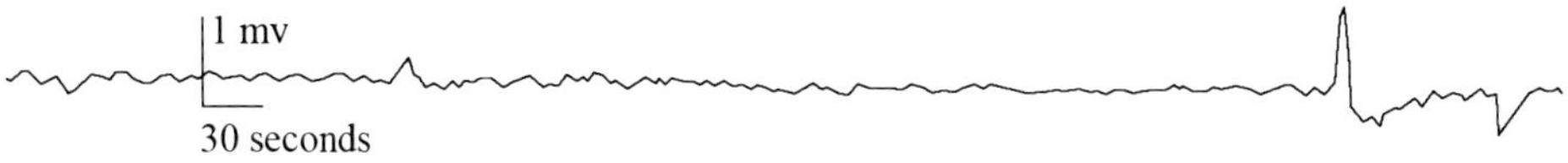

Figure 61. Two kinds of bioelectrical reactions recorded after stimulation of the Bonghan duct

In the experiments with the isolated specimen the earlier waves of low amplitudes are very difficult to recognize.

The earlier changes after the stimulation of the Bonghan duct are expressed usually as mono-phasic waves, while the later ones are mostly of high-potential spikes succeeded by prolonged positive after-potential.

The time needed for the manifestation of changes fluctuates widely, [p43] depending upon the intensity of the stimuli, the conditions of the Bonghan duct, especially upon the grade of its extension, and the temperature and humidity of the surrounding media; but it is generally proportional to the distance between the stimulating electrode and the recording electrode.

The velocity at which the first excitement is propagated, is estimated at about 1-3 mm per second.

The above facts reveal that there are two types of stimuli-effect in the Bonghan duct, i.e., one with swift and the other with slow propagation.

When the Bonghan duct of the abdominal aorta of a rabbit is stimulated and the electrical changes are recorded from the Bonghan duct of the caudal vena cava of the animal, or vice versa, all the effects in both cases bear similar character even though there is a slight difference of time needed for the manifestation of change.

This indicates that the effect can be transmitted to both directions in the Bonghan duct under experimental conditions.

3. Mechanical movement of Bonghan duct

Judging from the morphological structure and the bioelectrical changes, it seemed quite probable to us that the Bonghan duct might also make a certain kind of movements like the Bonghan corpuscle, so we studied the movements of the Bonghan duct using its isolated specimen.

An internal Bonghan duct was put into a damp chamber containing serum-saline solution, and the movements of the Bonghan duct were observed either with or without addition of drugs under the microscope installed in the thermostat at the temperature of 39°C.

The autonomic movements of the Bonghan duct can be observed under such conditions.

The mode of the movements of the Bonghan duct is very unique and different from those of other autonomic organs.

The autonomic movements of the Bonghan duct observed under the microscope are classified into:

1. The Incessant or Periodical Movement in the Longitudinal Direction,
2. The Quick, Trembling and Pulsating Movement in the Transversal Direction and [p44]
3. The Undulating Movement, the Mixed Form of the Above-mention Two Movements.

Each one of such movements is observed repeatedly at regular intervals depending upon the various conditions of experiment; and the commonest and ruling movement is the transversal one.

The movements of the isolated Bonghan duct are recognised at shorter intervals right after the isolation, but they gradually become rare with the lapse of time, the intervals sometimes reaching from 20 to 40 seconds or even longer. The movements of the isolated specimen can be maintained even longer than 30 minutes when the temperature and the media are favorable.

The movements of the Bonghan duct differ according to various factors and conditions.

If the temperature of the media is low (below 35°C) the movements are weakened or rarely observed. At this time, if the temperature of the media is raised up to 39°C, the Bonghan duct begins to move again.

Feeble or weakened movements of Bonghan duct can be revived by the drugs affecting the cholinergic system.

Movements in this case are principally transversal.

But the longitudinal or undulating movement can also be observed in accordance with the sort and dosage of the drugs and the conditions of the Bonghan duct.

The type and magnitude of the movements of the Bonghan duct just isolated are mostly dependent upon the conditions of the organism prior to isolation.

When the Bonghan liquor flows in the same direction as the blood, the direction of the movements of the unstimulated Bonghan duct in the isolated specimen coincides with that of blood circulation, whereas the stimulated Bonghan duct moves sometimes against the direction of blood circulation. In this case, the movements are not extended farther.

The movements of the Bonghan duct are also observed under the comparative microscope.

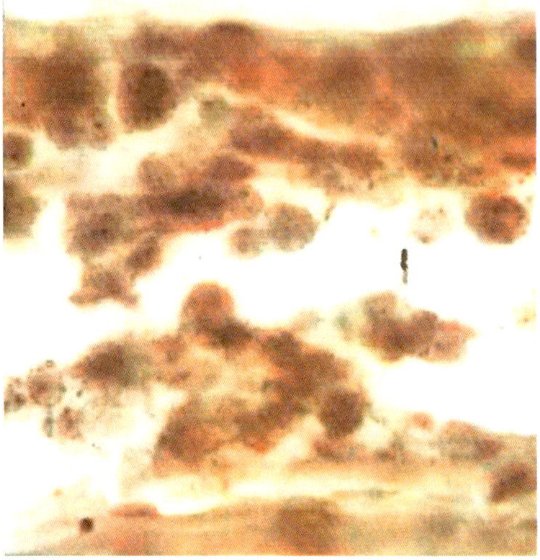

Figure 62. Microautoradiogram of the external Bonghan corpuscle
(2 hours after injection of P32 into the superficial Bonghan corpuscle) (x1,000)

The time needed for the recognition of the movements from one side to the other of the visual field was generally proportional to the distance between the two points concerned.

When the velocity of the movements of the Bonghan duct is measured by the above-mentioned method, it is estimated at about 0.1-0.6 mm/sec. The velocity depends mainly upon the conditions of the Bonghan duct and the intensity of the stimuli. [p45]

4. Relationship between bioelectrical changes and mechanical movements of Bonghan duct

Based on the fact that the Bonghan duct contracts autonomously and the definite bioelectrical changes appear in it, it is necessitated to explain the relationship between them.

Observing the movements of the Bonghan duct, the bioelectrical changes of the observed region were also recorded at the same time.

In this case, the movements of the Bonghan duct are preceded by bioelectrical changes for a definite period of time.

The electrical changes preceding the movements of the Bonghan duct are commonly exhibited as waves of longer periods and higher amplitudes. If the movements of the Bonghan duct are activated and made frequent by chemical stimuli, the preceding electrical changes are also intensified.

When the movements of the Bonghan duct are suppressed by chemical stimuli and made unnoticeable, the electrical changes are also weakened.

The movements of the Bonghan duct remain unnoticed, when comparatively quick electrical changes occur right after the stimulation; and later, when electrical changes of longer periods and higher amplitudes appear, the movements of the Bonghan duct are discerned. Sometimes faint electrical changes are recognized, even though the movements of the Bonghan duct are not noticeable.

These changes seem to be related to the movements of the individual Bonghan ductule.

III. Study on circulation of Bonghan liquor

Microautoradiography was applied for a more detailed study on the circulation of Bonghan liquor, an important biological function of the Kyungrak system. Radioisotopic disodium phosphate ($Na_2 HP^{32} O_4$) and dipotassium phosphate ($K_2 HP^{32} O_4$) were used and nuclear emulsion NUC-715 was smeared for radioautography.

To examine the process of the circulation of Bonghan liquor, particularly the correlations between the various systems of Kyungrak, isotopes in the quantity of 100-200 μC were injected into various positions of the Kyungrak system, and specimens from various parts of the [p46] Kyungrak system and from different tissues were taken at the intervals of 10 and 30 minutes, 2, 12 and 28 hours after the injection and were microautoradiographed. In order to study the circulation of Bonghan liquor in the external Bonghan duct system, radioactive phosphorus (P32) was injected into a superficial Bonghan corpuscle; then external Bonghan corpuscles in the neck and abdomen were microautoradiographed.

It was ascertained that the Bonghan ductules in the external Bonghan corpuscles and the nuclei of chromaffine cells, pale nuclei, round nucleus-like structures, and basophile granules began to be labelled in two hours after the injection (Figure 62).

But P32 was to be detected neither in the blood elements inside the blood vessels of these corpuscles nor in the connective tissues surrounding them.

P32 injected into the ear vein could hardly be traced in the external Bonghan corpuscle. Nevertheless, P32 injected into the external Bonghan corpuscle of the neck was seen in the internal Bonghan duct, but not in the superficial Bonghan corpuscle (Figure 63).

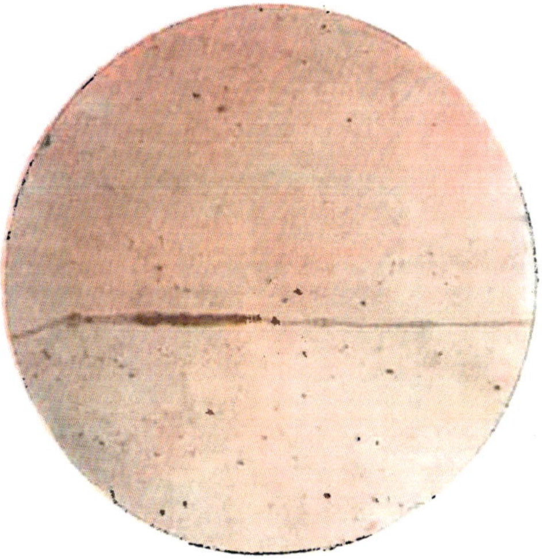

Figure 63. Microautoradiogram of the internal Bonghan duct
(3 hours after injection of P32 into the superficial Bonghan corpuscle) (x160)

The findings tell us that the Bonghan liquor flows between the superficial and the external Bonghan corpuscle, and that it circulates only in one direction from the superficial to the profund Bonghan corpuscle.

In order to clarify the correlations between the external and the internal Bonghan duct and the circulation of the Bonghan liquor within them, P32 was injected into an internal Bonghan duct, and then the superficial and the external Bonghan corpuscle were microautoradiographed.

The elements of the inner substance of the superficial Bonghan corpuscle were tagged and P32 was observed between the smooth muscle cells in the outer layer in three hours after the injection (Figure 64), but the isotope was rarely recognized in the connective tissues surrounding the Bonghan corpuscles.

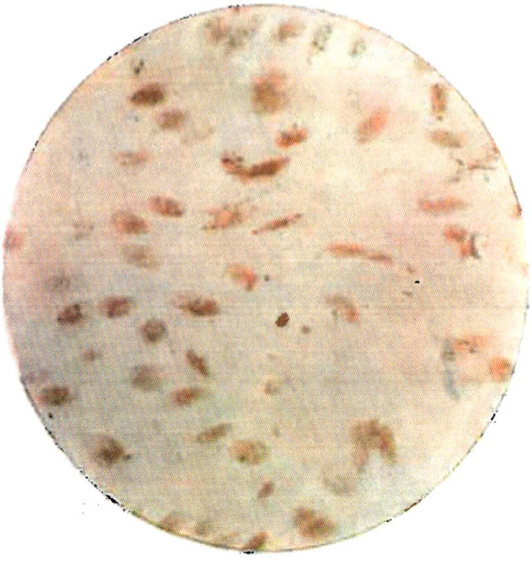

Figure 64. Microautoradiogram of the superficial Bonghan corpuscle
(3 hours after injection of P32 into the internal Bonghan duct) (x400)

The results of the injection of P32 into external Bonghan corpuscles were the same as in the case of superficial Bonghan corpuscles (Figure 65).

When P32 is injected into the superficial and external Bonghan corpuscles, and internal Bonghan ducts in the blood vessels are observed three hours later, P32 is found in one or several ductules. In some cases, nuclei of endothelial and outer membrane cells are tagged. A lot of P32 is often seen in some positions of the ductule, where the ductules look bulged, which implies the contraction of the Bonghan ducts. The constituent parts in the internal Bonghan corpuscle are also labelled.

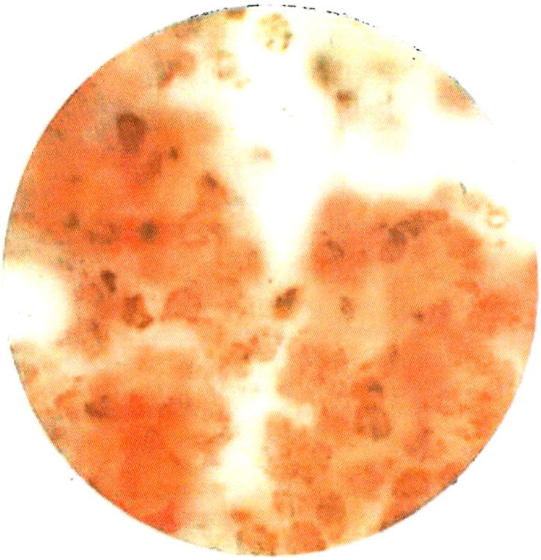

Figure 65. Microautoradiogram of the external Bonghan corpuscle
(3 hours after injection of P32 into the internal Bonghan duct) (x400)

Table 7. Results of injection of 200 μC of P32 (after 6 hours)

Locus of injection	Organ examined	Total number of cells observed	Number of labelled cells	Percentage
External Bonghan corpuscle	Ovary	17,850	78	0.437
Internal Bonghan corpuscle	Ovary	19,525	42	0.214
Ear vein	Ovary	21,633	7	0.032

This proves that the circulation of Bonghan liquor in the internal Bonghan duct and in the external Bonghan duct is linked with each other. [p47]

In order to study the peripheral circulation of Bonghan liquor P32 was injected into the circulating systems of the internal and external Bonghan ducts, and various internal organs were examined.

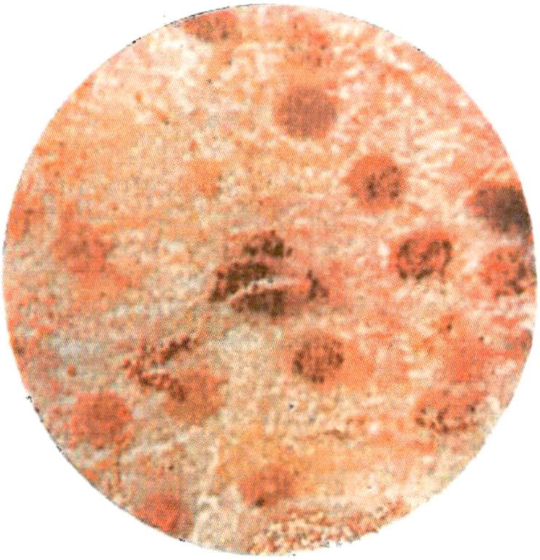

Figure 66. Microautoradiogram of the ovary (6 hours after injection of P32 into the superficial Bonghan corpuscle) (x1,000)

It has been disclosed that cortical and medullary cells of the ovary were labelled in 6 hours after the injection (Figure 66).

Table 7 shows the number of labelled cells in comparison with the case of injection of P32 into a blood vessel.

In some cases, one can see no distinct Bonghan ductules but recognize only a line of P32, reaching a labelled nucleus.

Particular mention should be made of the fact that when P32 is injected into a superficial Bonghan corpuscle, it concentrates on the nuclei of a certain part of the ovary. When P32 is injected into the internal Bonghan duct and the liver is observed (after 6 hours), as shown in Table 8, most of P32 is to be seen in the nuclei of the parenchymal cells of the liver and very few in the epithelial cells of biliary ducts and Kupffer cells.

Table 8. Results of the injection of 200 μC of P32 (after 6 hours)

Position of P32 injection	Organs observed	Total number of cells observed	Number of labelled cells	Percentage
Internal Bonghan duct	Liver	17,805	34	0.190
Ear vein	Liver	21,638	4	0.018

The above-mentioned results accord with the morphological findings of the intraorganic system of Kyungrak.

Especially noteworthy is the confirmation of P32 in the cell nuclei, [p48] which coincides with the histological finding that the terminal Bonghan ductules reach cell nuclei.

When dyes, instead of isotopes, are injected into the Bonghan duct, they are also observed only in the nuclei of cells.

In the liver, dyes appear mainly in the nuclei of parenchymal cells and rarely in the nuclei of Kupffer cells and of epithelial cells of biliary ducts. In this case, terminal

Bonghan ductules connected with the cells are also stained.

IV. Effect of stimuli to Bonghan duct

The influences of the stimuli to a Bonghan duct upon the heart function, movements of the intestines and upon the contraction of the skeletal muscle were studied.

1. Influence of stimuli to Bonghan duct on heart function

An internal Bonghan duct of a rabbit was stimulated and its electrocardiogram was studied. Bonghan ducts, chiefly in the artery and vein of cervical and femoral regions, were stimulated with drugs.

Changes take place in the heart function some time after the stimulus is given to an internal Bonghan duct. This change is mainly manifested in either increase or decrease of the heart beat.

About 46 per cent of the positive cases show the changes in the force of cardiac contraction. This is related with the kind of the stimulating drugs used and the conditions of the animal at the time of stimulation.

However, weaker effects were observed in general when the femoral blood vessels were stimulated than in case of the affection of the carotid blood vessels.

The change in the number of heart beat precedes that in the force of heart beat by one or two minutes. The increase in the number of heart beat is accompanied by lower amplitude and the decrease in it by higher amplitude.

These results show that the stimuli given to the internal Bonghan duct exert their influence first on the rhythm of the heart function and then on the contraction of the heart. Stimuli given to the Bonghan duct bring forth changes in the number of beating, amplitude and wave [p49] pattern of the heart in two phases generally.

The changes in the first phase are generally inferior to those in the second phase in their magnitude and duration.

The interval between these two phases is proportional to the distance of the stimulated locus from the heart.

And in case of applying stimuli to the Bonghan duct in the artery, the time needed for the manifestation of the changes fluctuates in a very wide range.

In view of the sluggish propagation of the movements of the Bonghan duct, we consider that the first phase of the changes caused by the stimuli given to the Bonghan duct indicates the earlier effects of these stimuli and has nothing to do with the propagation of the movements of the Bonghan duct, whereas the second phase corresponds to the movements of the Bonghan duct.

The fact that the effect of the stimuli given to the Bonghan duct in the artery appears later and the time needed for the manifestation of changes varies more sharply than in the case of the vein, suggests that the direction of the movements of the Bonghan duct in that case is opposite to the blood circulation.

2. Influence of stimuli to Bonghan duct on movements of the intestines

The movements of the intestines of a rabbit were either recorded by means of suspending in situ or watched on the abdominal wall, when drugs were applied to the Bonghan ducts in femoral blood vessels.

Such a stimulus brings about changes in the movements of the intestines after a definite span of time.

The patterns of the changes vary according to the loci of the stimuli.

When stimuli are applied to the Bonghan duct in the femoral vein the frequency of contraction increases and the tonus elevates, and, at the same time, the force of contraction increases generally. When stimuli are given to the Bonghan duct in the femoral artery, the force of contraction generally weakens with its increasing frequency, and there is rare increase either in the force of contraction or in tonus.

After the stimulation of an internal Bonghan duct follow the repeated changes in the movements of the intestines. Study of these changes reveals that among the effects of the stimuli given to the internal Bonghan duct upon the movements of the intestines there are effects of stimuli which propagate more swiftly than the movements of the duct. [p50]

3. Influence of stimuli to Bonghan duct on the contraction of skeletal muscle

While recording the ergogram of a slightly loaded gastrocnemius of either a rabbit or a frog through the stimulation of the sciatic nerve with induction current (60 stimuli per minute for the rabbit and 50 per minute for the frog), the Bonghan duct was stimulated.

To the Bonghan duct in the artery of one side were applied drugs, and the ergograms were recorded each time right after, and one and three minutes after the stimulation. And then the maximal mean contraction degree, the time of fatigue needed for the initial contraction degree to be reduced to its half value, and the area covered by the ergogram were estimated.

The mean ergogram thus recorded at definite intervals after the stimulation of the internal Bonghan duct of a rabbit is shown in Figure 67.

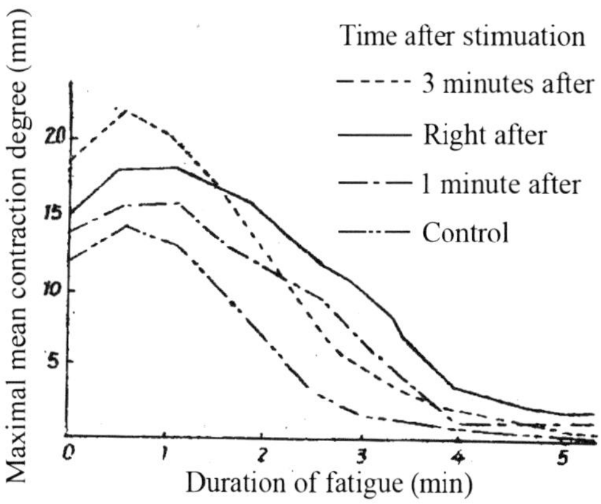

Figure 67. Ergogram of the skeletal muscle recorded after the stimulation of the internal Bonghan duct at definite intervals

As is shown in Fig. 14, it is clear that the mean contraction degree, the duration of fatigue, and the area occupied by the ergogram of the experimental animals are surpassing those of the control animals (Table 9). [p51]

Table 9. Changes or ergogram following the stimulation of an internal Bonghan duct

Time elapsed after stimulation	Maximal mean contraction degree (mm)	Time needed for initial contraction degree to drop by 50% (sec)	Area covered by ergogram (cm^2)
Control	13	120	10.15
Right after	19	195	17.00
1 minute after	16	173	17.00
3 minutes after	22	144	15.60

According to this Table, the maximal mean contraction degree is the highest in the case recorded three minutes after the stimulation and the time needed for the 50 per cent reduction of the initial contraction degree is the longest in the case recorded right after the stimulation.

Wider area of ergogram and longer time of fatigue were observed, when recording was done either right after or one minute after the stimulation.

Such experiments were also carried out on frogs and the results obtained were quite the same as in the case of rabbits. These phenomena, we believe, have a certain relationship with the sluggish propagation of the effect of the stimuli given to the Bonghan duct. In this connection, further explanation can be given as follows:

In case that the recording is started three minutes after the stimulation the initial contraction degree is high but the time of fatigue and the area of ergogram are not much, since the effect of a stimulus on the Bonghan duct has already reached the gastrocnemius prior to the registration. However, when the recordings were done both right after and one minute after the stimulation, the contraction degree remains in lower niveau and the duration of fatigue becomes longer and the area of the ergogram larger. This suggests that the effect of the stimulus has already reached the gastrocnemius by the time when the skeletal muscle begins to get tired.

This opinion is supported by the experiments on frogs: the fatigue time of the skeletal muscle appears later when the Bonghan duct is stimulated a minute after the outset of the recording than in the case of the recording right after the stimulation (Figure 68). [p52]

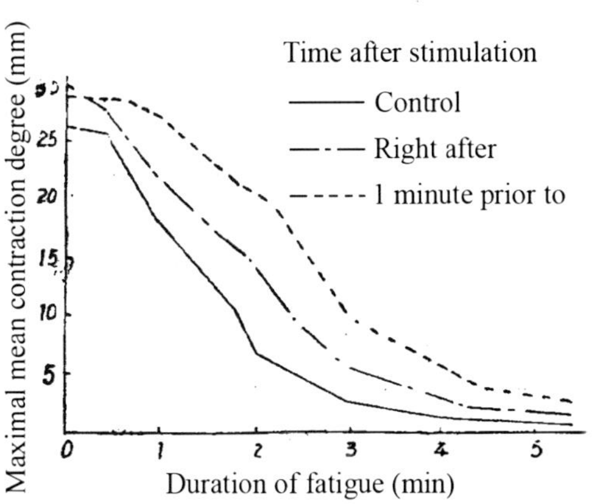

Figure 68. Comparison of the ergogram recorded right after stimulation of the internal Bonghan duct to that recorded 1 minute prior to stimulation

When the sciatic nerve of a frog is stimulated at the rate of 50 frequencies per minute, the fatigue curve of the gastrocnemius shows that the muscle is in a state of isometrical contraction.

The magnitude of the isometrical muscular contractions in the experimental and control groups is compared in Figure 69. [p53]

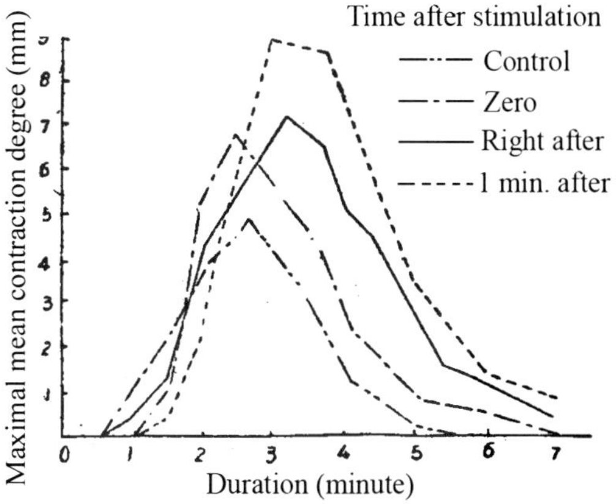

Figure 69. Changes of the isometrical muscle contraction following stimulation of the internal Bonghan duct

As is seen in Fig. 16, the intensity of isometrical muscular contraction is generally more accentuated in the experimental group than in the control group. And in the experimental group the intensity of contraction gradually increases in the following order: the case of stimulation one minute after the outset of the recording, that of recording right after the stimulation and that of the recording one minute after the stimulation; and in the last case the intensity doubles that of the control group.

The above-mentioned experimental data show that the stimulation given to the Bonghan duct not only delays the appearance of the fatigue process by giving a definite influence on the contraction of skeletal muscle and increases the activity of muscle, but also enhances the tonus of skeletal muscle.

V. Effect of cutting of Bonghan duct

To clarify the relations between the Kyungrak and the nervous system, the influence on the spinal reflex as well as on the excitability of the peripheral nerve caused by the cutting of the perineurial Bonghan duct was examined.

1. Influence on spinal reflex time

Having estimated the time of bending reflex of the leg of a spinal frog by stimulating with 0.5 per cent solution of sulfuric acid, we repeated the same experiment at different intervals—30 minutes, 12, 24, 36 and 48 hours—after the cutting of the perineurial Bonghan duct and compared the results with each other.

The reflex time in all cases of the severed perineurial Bonghan duct was lengthened.

Figure 70 indicates the mean reflex time of the experimental and the control group. The abscissa represents the number of repetition and the ordinate the reflex time in seconds (Figure 70).

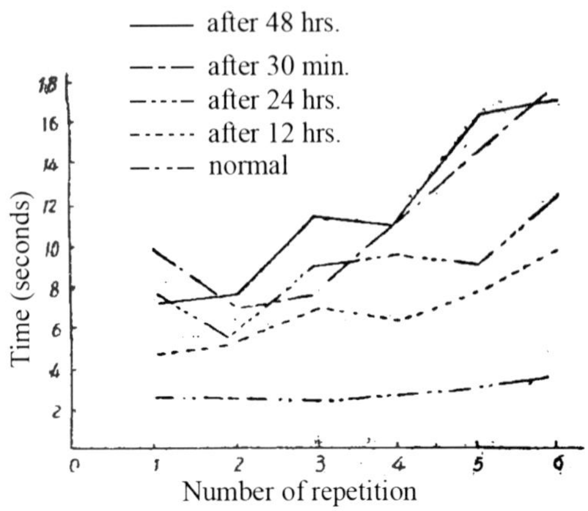

Figure 70. Changes of spinal reflex time measured at intervals after cutting the Bonghan duct according to the number of repetition of the experiment

As is shown in Fig. 17, the reflex time of the experimental group fluctuates in a wider range, depending on the number of repetition, with the tendency of being lengthened. [p54]

The mean reflex time of every six experiments on the experimental and the control group is shown in Table 10.

Table 10. Changes of spinal reflex time after cutting Bonghan duct

No.	Time after cutting	Avg reflex time (sec) based on 6 experiments	Control
1	Normal	2.5	—
2	30 min	11.5	2.5
3	12 hours	6.3	2.3
4	24 hours	8.7	3.0
5	36 hours	10.3	3.0
6	48 hours	11.3	3.1

This Table shows that the reflex time sharply lengthens in 30 minutes after the cutting, and soon recovers, then gradually lengthens with the lapse of time.

The experimental data mentioned above bespeak that the perineurial Bonghan ducts exert a certain influence on the spinal reflex and this influence intensifies as time passes after the cutting of the Bonghan duct.

The fact that the reflex time after the cutting of a Bonghan duct [p55] fluctuates markedly according to the number of repetition also indicates that the spinal reflex becomes very unstable.

Histological examinations of the nerve fibres in the region of the severed Bonghan duct were carried out at definite intervals. Histological changes were observed in the myelin sheath and axon 12 hours after the cutting. These changes are not limited to the severed locus of the Bonghan duct. The histological changes reach the remote distal region.

This means that the Kyungrak system exerts a certain trophic influence upon the nervous system.

2. Influence on excitability of peripheral nerves

A perineurial Bonghan duct of a frog was cut off for the purpose of examining the influence of the excitability of the peripheral nerves.

In order to cut off the perineurial Bonghan duct in the peripheral region of the sciatic nerve, perineurium was removed in the length of 7 mm, and then the remaining part of the nerve with perineurium was stimulated, and the threshold was estimated so as to compared it with that of a normal nerve. The threshold was estimated by the distance between the induction coils. The threshold of about 40-50 per cent of the affected cases showed a very high value.

The femoral region of the sciatic nerve was divided into three equal parts, and the perineurium of each part was removed successively, and the threshold of each case was determined. The values obtained reveal that the rise of the threshold is independent of the locus affected but is dependent upon the length of the removed perineurium.

When the whole perineurium of the sciatic nerve is removed, the rise of the threshold was observed in 70-80 per cent of the cases concerned.

When no change in the threshold was noticed by the removal of the perineurium in the lowest region of the sciatic nerve then the perineurium of the middle one-third part was removed, and if, nevertheless, the threshold remained unchanged, then the perineurium of the proximal one-third region was further taken off.

Such a successive removal of perineurium brought forth a gradual rise of the threshold in many cases.

Removal of the perineurium accompanies a remarkable rise in the threshold of nerves, whereas the threshold of the muscle remains unchanged.

And even when the muscle does not contract at the stimulus given [p56] to a proximal point of the nerve without perineurium, an action current, though feeble in amplitude, may also be observed at the distal region of the nerve deprived of perineurium.

These findings suggest that there exists a Bonghan duct in the perineurium.

3. Changes in innervation of muscles by motor nerves

Based on the fact that the perineurial Bonghan duct exerts a certain influence on the excitability of the peripheral nerves, the role of the Bonghan duct among the nerve fibres in the innervation of muscles by motor nerves was examined.

When the proximal nerve trunk of a single neurogastrocnemial specimen of a frog or a toad is stimulated, muscle contraction occurs merely in about 30 per cent of the cases.

In the case of the occurrence of muscle contraction, the time of its continuation was measured. The duration of muscle contraction was, in an absolute majority of the cases, less than an hour and only a few of the cases showed one to six hour contraction.

When examined histologically, only the single nerve fibre could be seen in the former case, while the neural Bonghan ductule around the nerve fibre was additionally found in the latter case.

This fact implies that the neural Bonghan duct plays an important role in the innervation of muscles by motor nerves.

It has been also established that when the sciatic perineurium of a rabbit is stripped off, then "trophic ulcer" appears in its hind leg and degeneration occurs in the nerve fibre itself.

All these experiments indicate that the Kyungrak system not only exerts an influence on the nervous system, but also directly participates in muscle contraction, as well as in the trophic innervation of muscles by nerves.

VI. Path of circulation of Bonghan liquor

The Bonghan liquor circulates inside the Bonghan duct. As stated above, Kyungrak has various systems of Bonghan ducts. But the Bonghan liquor does not circulate through a single system. It is considered [p57] that the circulation course of the Bonghan liquor is a closed one, running through the different systems along diversely connected paths.

On the basis of anatomico-histological and physiological experimental data on the Kyungrak system, particularly the findings obtained by means of radioisotopes, we can suggest the scheme of the path of circulation of the Bonghan liquor as seen in Figure 71.

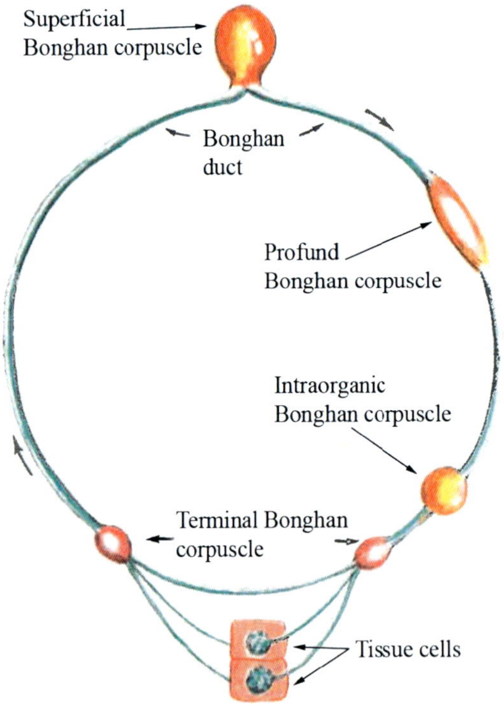

Figure 71. Scheme of the circulation route of the Bonghan liquor

The scheme aims to illustrate the following features:

1. All tissue cells are situated on the closed path of circulation of the Bonghan liquor.

2. Every organism has not only one but many such courses of circulation which are intricately linked with each other.

3. A circulation course should always go through: Tissue cells—superficial Bonghan corpuscle—profund Bonghan corpuscle—intraorganic Bonghan corpuscle—terminal Bonghan corpuscle—tissue cells.

4. Communication between the Bonghan corpuscles can be maintained by one to three of the following ducts: internal Bonghan duct, external Bonghan duct, neural Bonghan duct and intra-external Bonghan duct.

5. The terminal corpuscle is linked with a certain number of tissue cells. [p58]

Part IV. Embryological and comparative biologic studies on Kyungrak system

1. Embryological studies on the Kyungrak system

In the embryological research in the Kyungrak system, we started from clarifying the primordium of the Bonghan duct and its stage of differentiation.

In order to make clear the development of the Bonghan duct, systematic observations were made on the chick embryos incubated for different lengths of time.

Between the ectoderm and yolk sac of the chick embryo before incubation, basophile granules are found lying freely, and they are also arranged between blastodermic cells.

In the chick embryo incubated for 5 hours' these basophile granules are scattered or amassed, and sometimes are arranged regularly.

In the chick embryo of seven to eight hours' incubation mesoderm begins to differentiate, and at this time peculiar cells distinguishable from those of mesoderm appear between the ectoderm and the entoderm of the pellucid area and the opaque area.

The shape of these cells is elongated ellipsoidal and small processes protrude at their both ends, reminding one of a bipolar cell, and their cytoplasm is filled with fine and coarse basophile granules. The nucleus of such cell is oval and located in the centre of the cell body.

These particular cells are called the primitive cells of the Bonghan duct, as the Bonghan duct develops from these cells.

In the embryo of 10 hours' incubation the primitive cells of the Bonghan duct, being arranged in a definite direction, form syncytium [p59] connected with one another by their cytoplasmic processes. In the syncytium, basophile granules can be seen and the nucleus, oval in shape, is located in the centre of the cell body. The syncytial structures of these primitive cells differentiate and develop to form the Bonghan duct. So they are regarded as the primordium of the duct.

In the embryo of 10 hours' incubation the primitive cells of the duct differentiates rapidly and begins to change remarkably.

The primitive cells of the Bonghan duct lose their boundary and form a cord-like structure, in the centre of which are located ellipsoidal nuclei, and the cell membrane forms the wall of the Bonghan duct. This structure is considered to be the primitive Bonghan duct.

The fact that the Bonghan duct, with the basically-completed tubular structure, develops in the embryo of 10-15 hours' incubation, in which primordia of organs are not yet differentiated, suggests that the function of the Kyungrak system, in the light of its role in the adult, exerts an influence upon the differentiation of cells, organogenesis and histogenesis of organism.

In the embryo of 20 hours' incubation, the primitive Bonghan duct continuously differentiates and develops through the pellucid area into the opaque area. At this time mesenchymal cells differentiated from mesoderm are amassed in the opaque area and, surrounding the primitive

Bonghan duct, bring into shape a blood island. It is quite probable that the Bonghan liquor flowing in the Bonghan duct promotes and completes the formation of the blood island and blood vessels.

The oval nuclei of the primitive Bonghan duct are gradually elongated to become rod-shaped, migrate from the centre of the primitive duct to its wall and develop into endothelial nuclei of the Bonghan duct.

Thus the Bonghan ductules are formed. From the blood island around the completed Bonghan ductules, blood vessels begin to take shape and in the embryo incubated for 20-27 hours these Bonghan ductules are surrounded with blood vessels and develop into the internal Bonghan duct. New Bonghan ductules are formed during the period of 20-27 to 48 hours of incubation and the differentiation and development of the newly formed ductules are the same as the already completed Bonghan ductules.

The ductules formed in the embryo incubated for 20-27 hours, together with those formed subsequently, make up a bundle and develop into a Bonghan duct. Therefore, in the embryo incubated for 45 hours to 5 days, various stages of formation of the Bonghan duct can be seen.

As we have seen, the Bonghan duct not only develops earlier but also completes differentiation and formation more rapidly than the blood vessels and nerves. [p60]

The process of formation of the Bonghan duct, being different from that of the blood and lymphatic vessels, includes the following stages: the stage of the primitive cell of the Bonghan duct (incubated for 7-8 hours), stage of the primordium of the Bonghan duct (incubated for 10 hours), stage of the primitive Bonghan duct (incubated for 15 hours), stage of completing the Bonghan ductules (incubated for 20-28 hours), stage of formation of the Bonghan duct (incubated for 27-48 hours), and stage of completing the Bonghan duct (incubated for 48 hours).

Noteworthy is the fact that such basophile granules as are visible in the Bonghan duct are also proved in the chick embryo of the earliest stage of its development.

2. Comparative biological studies on the Kyungrak system

The results of the embryological studies on the Kyungrak system suggest that this system develops very early phylogenetically.

We confirmed the existence of the Kyungrak system not only in the mammals but also in the Aves, Reptilia, Amphibia and Pisces. The structures of the Bonghan ducts of these animals are little different from one another, but the endothelial nuclei of the ducts of the other animals are larger and clearer than those of the mammals. The structures of the Bonghan corpuscles are simpler, and cells with pale cytoplasm and basophile structures are amassed in the corpuscles.

The Kyungrak system is also present in the invertebrates. In the coelenteron of the hydra which belongs to the coelenterate runs the Bonghan duct and its branches are distributed in the ectoderm and the entoderm.

The Kyungrak system is considered to exist in all the multi-cellular animals.

The Kyungrak system exists not only in the animal but also in the vegetable kingdom. [p61]

Conclusion

I. Kyungrak Consists of Several Systems

A. All the Systems Are Composed of Bonghan Ducts and Bonghan Corpuscles with Common Structures.

All the Bonghan Corpuscles Are Linked by Bonghan Ducts with One Another.

All the Bonghan Ducts Connect the Bonghan Corpuscles With One Another.

The Bonghan Duct Is Formed of a Bundle Which Consists of One to Scores of Bonghan Ductules.

1. The Bonghan ductule is formed of thin endothelial cells with peculiar rod-shaped nuclei and has an outer membrane composed of smooth muscle-like cells and fine argyrophile fibres.

Fibrous structures and amorphous substance are found between Bonghan ductules.

A number of Bonghan ductules are bound in a bundle by a periductium.

The periductium has its own cells.

The Bonghan ductule contains basophile granules and small nucleus-like structures.

2. The Bonghan corpuscle is mainly formed of the dilated, ramified and anastomosed Bonghan ductules.

At the same time the reticular elements of the outer membrane, interstitial substance of the Bonghan ductule and the periductium constitute the main structural components of the Bonghan corpuscle.

The enlarged Bonghan duct sinus contains cell elements and chromaffine granules as well as basophile structures. [p62]

B. Following Are the Different Systems of Kyungrak:

1. The Internal Bonghan Duct System

It consists of internal Bonghan ducts and internal Bonghan corpuscles and is distributed systematically and consecutively in all the blood vessels, lymphatic vessels and the cardiac cavity.

The internal Bonghan duct is extremely fragile and its periductium and interstitial substance are poorly developed.

The internal Bonghan corpuscle has a structure remarkably resembling to that of the hematopoietic organ, and myeloid and lymphoid cells are found in the network of the reticular tissues.

An assemblage of cells similar to those of a number of parenchymal organs are also found sometimes.

2. The Intra-external Bonghan Duct System

It consists of intra-external Bonghan ducts and intra-external Bonghan corpuscles and runs independently of the surrounding organs and of the blood and lymphatic vessels and nerves.

In the intra-external Bonghan duct interstitial substance and periductium are more developed than in the internal Bonghan duct.

The Bonghan duct sinus of the intra-external Bonghan corpuscle contains cells with pale cytoplasm as well as basophile structures.

3. The External Bonghan Duct System

It consists of external Bonghan ducts and external Bonghan corpuscles and mainly runs around vessels and nerves. Thick connective tissue membrane covers the external Bonghan duct.

The Bonghan duct sinus of the external Bonghan corpuscle contains a lot of chromaffine granules.

4. The Neural Bonghan Duct System

It consists of neural Bonghan ducts and neural Bonghan corpuscles and floats in the cerebrospinal fluid of the central nervous system.

Its branches are distributed not only in the parenchyma of the central nervous system but also in the peripheral nerves.

5. The Intraorganic System of Kyungrak

In the organs, too, there are distributed intraorganic Bonghan [p63] corpuscles, terminal Bonghan corpuscles and terminal Bonghan ductules.

They are the intraorganic parts of the internal Bonghan ducts, external Bonghan ducts and neural Bonghan ducts.

Various Bonghan ducts are merged in the intraorganic Bonghan corpuscle to become terminal Bonghan ductules, which are linked directly with cell nuclei. Fine Bonghan ductules again come out from the tissue cells.

Different systems of Kyungrak are linked with one another. The internal Bonghan duct system communicates with the intra-external Bonghan duct system through the blood vessel wall and with the external Bonghan duct system through the external Bonghan corpuscles.

The intra-external Bonghan duct system communicates with the external Bonghan duct system through the external Bonghan corpuscles and is linked with the neural Bonghan duct system.

All the systems are intimately related with one another.

II. The Kyungrak System Is the Multi-circulation System of Bonghan Liquor

A. The Biochemical Composition of Bonghan Liquor is As Follows:

It contains a great deal of DNA and RNA.

The total amount of nitrogen accounts for 3.12 - 3.40 per cent and that of nonprotein nitrogen 0.10 - 0.17 per cent. Lipid amounts to 0.57 - 1.00 per cent and reduced sugar 0.10 - 0.12 per cent.

The total amount of hyaluronic acid is estimated at 170.4 mg/%.

20 kinds of free amino acids, including essential amino acid, are found.

No less than 16 kinds of free mononucleotides are present.

B. The Bonghan Duct Shows Bioelectrical Activity As Well As Conductibility of Stimuli and Motility.

1. The electrical changes in the Bonghan duct are very slow and are nearly similar to the "ㄱ" and "ㄴ" waves that can be observed in the Bonghan corpuscle. These electrical changes appear in different pat-

terns when stimuli are given to the Bonghan duct. [p64]

2. Bioelectrical changes are transmitted, along the Bonghan duct when it is stimulated. The electrical changes of low amplitude are transmitted rapidly (1 - 3 mm/sec.) and those of high amplitude slowly.

3. The Bonghan duct makes autonomic movement. This movement is propagated and it changes when the Bonghan duct is stimulated. There are different patterns of movement of the Bonghan duct continuous or periodical longitudinal movement and vibrating transversal movement. These data support the fact that the Bonghan duct ensures conditions for the active circulation of Bonghan liquor.

C. All the Tissue Cells Are Directly Connected with the Kyungrak System.

1. All the tissue cells are furnished with fine terminal Bonghan ductules penetrating into cell nuclei and coming out of them.

These ductules are linked with intraorganic Bonghan corpuscles.

Each Intraorganic Bonghan corpuscle is linked only with the tissue cells of a definite range.

2. The intraorganic Bonghan corpuscles are linked with all the systems of Kyungrak, that is, the different systems of Kyungrak start from the intraorganic Bonghan corpuscles and end in the intraorganic Bonghan corpuscles.

D. Following Are the Results of the Observations on the Paths of Bonghan Liquor after the Injection of Radioactive Phosphorus (P32) into Various Parts of the Kyungrak System.

The Bonghan liquor flowing from various organs and tissues is considered to be circulating towards the superficial Bonghan corpuscles.

The Bonghan liquor starting from the superficial Bonghan corpuscles reaches the profund Bonghan corpuscles.

The Bonghan liquor flowing from the profund Bonghan corpuscles reaches tissue cells through the intraorganic Bonghan corpuscles. The same results are obtained in the experiments by stain injection too.

E. The Circulating Courses of Bonghan Liquor Are Not Unitary.

The circulating courses of Bonghan liquor, unlike the course of blood circulation, are not unitary but are many, and they are interlinked, [p65] while maintaining relative independence.

The stain or isotope injected into a circulating course of Bonghan liquor circulates only in a certain limited region.

But the Bonghan liquor moves sometimes from one circulating course to another through the routes linking them together.

III. The Changes in the Circulation of the Bonghan Liquor Exert Influence on the Functions of Different Organs

A. The Stimulation to the Bonghan Duct Affects the Number of Heart Beat and the Force of Cardiac Con-

traction and Brings About Changes in the Movements of the Intestines.

And It Exerts Tangible Influence on the Ergogram of the Skeletal Muscle.

B. When the Bonghan Duct Is Cut, Marked Changes Are Noticed in the Tissue Cells.

When the Bonghan duct is cut, karyolysis occurs in the tissue cells connected to it, and the cells die.

When the Bonghan duct of the peripheral nerve is cut, the excitability of the nerve decreases remarkably.

When the Bonghan duct of the motor nerve is cut and repeated stimulation is given to this nerve, the muscle ceases to contract within a short span of time.

IV. The Differentiation and Development of the Kyungrak System Precede the Differentiations of the Vascular and Nervous Systems and Other Organs

In the chick embryo the development of the Bonghan ductule passes the stage of the primitive cell of the Bonghan duct after 7-8 hours' incubation, the primordial stage of the Bonghan duct after 10 hours' incubation, the stage of the primitive Bonghan ductule after 15 hours' incubation, and the stage of completion after 20-28 hours' incubation. [p66]

The precedence of the differentiation and development of the Kyungrak system suggests the role of this system in the embryonic development of organisms.

V. The Kyungrak System Is Considered To Be Existing Widely in the Biological World

The Kyungrak system is found not only in the mammals but also in other vertebrates and invertebrates. It exists in plants as well. It is considered that this system finds itself in all the multi-cellular organisms.

According to the findings about the Kyungrak system, the circulating course of the Bonghan liquor is as follows:

The tissue cell—the superficial Bonghan corpuscle—the profund Bonghan corpuscle—the intraorganic Bonghan corpuscle—the terminal Bonghan corpuscle—the tissue cell.

The Kyungrak system is a multi-circulating system in which the paths of circulation of the Bonghan liquor are interlinked and integrated.

All the morphological constituent parts of an organism are connected with the Kyungrak system and are arranged in good order along the Kyungrak system.

To say, every organism is considered to have the system of Kyungrak. [p67]

THEORY OF SANAL

INTRODUCTION

In the course of studying the physiological functions of the Kyungrak system, a new anatomico-histological system in the organism, we have come to realize the new important facts which underlie all the phenomena of life. We have ascertained that unique granules (they are named "Bonghan sanal" after the discoverer) circulate in the Kyungrak system and they grow into cells, and that the cells of organs and tissues turn into the Bonghan sanal, while moving through the Kyungrak system.

This process is repeated in a continuous cycle. (This cyclic process is called "Bonghan sanal-cell cycle").

Through the research into the continuous process of the "Bonghan sanal-cell cycle," we have come to form the following new views on the self-renovation of the organism.

All the Morphological Constituent Parts of the Organism Are Incessantly Renewed.

The Self-renovation of the Organism Takes the Form of "Bonghan Sanal-Cell Cycle."

The Self-renovation of the Organism Is Performed by the Kyungrak System.

We name these views "Theory of Sanal." A series of researches have been performed to prove the validity of these views. Results obtained are presented here.

The theory of sanal, of course, requires the re-examination of the cell theory and other cardinal problems of biology. [p69]

Chapter I. Circulation in the Kyungrak system

In explaining the physiological functions of the Kyungrak system, the first question to be answered is what kind of role does Bonghan liquor play during its circulation in the Kyungrak system.

To get answer for this question, it is necessary, in the first place, to examine the course of circulation and composition of the Bonghan liquor.

I. Circulation course of Bonghan liquor

The circulation course of Bonghan liquor is not unitary like that of blood circulation. Each part of the organs is linked to a relevant circulating route. The circulating routes are interrelated.

The circulation course of Bonghan liquor begins from cells and ends in cells. The courses pass through the superficial and profund Bonghan corpuscles. These characteristics of the circulation course of Bonghan liquor raise important questions on the function and role of the Kyungrak system.

II. Contents of Bonghan liquor

The striking feature of the composition of Bonghan liquor is that it contains a large amount of nucleic and, DNA in particular (cf. "On the Kyungrak system," Proceedings of the Academy of Medical Sciences, D.P.R.K., No 5, Nov. 30, 1963).

Bonghan liquor is also rich in RNA, protein and free amino acids.

Besides these, it has sugar and lipids along with adrenocortical [p70] hormone, adrenomedullary hormone, sex hormone, mononucleotides and much hyaluronic acid. Clarification of the biological significance of these contents of Bonghan liquor is of major importance in explicating the function of the Kyungrak system. Bonghan liquor has many granular structures which show positive Feulgen reaction. These granular structures have various forms and sizes from a small granule measuring about 0.8 micron in diameter to a large one measuring 5-10 microns. Several granules sticking together are also found. These granular structures were observed in living conditions under the phase contrast microscope for the clarification of their physiological significance.

As these granular structures grow into cells, they are named "Bonghan sanal."

When Feulgen test was performed on Bonghan sanal in each of the stages of its growth, Feulgen positive granular structures of various sizes and forms were observed just as in the Feulgen test on the Bonghan liquor.

Chapter II. Characteristics of sanal

I. Morphological characteristics of sanal

1. Methods of isolation and observation of sanal

As sanal exist in the Bonghan liquor, the liquor must, first of all, be drawn out of a Bonghan duct or of a Bonghan corpuscle to get sanal.

The Bonghan liquor is drawn out by puncturing a duct or a corpuscle with a fine glass capillary fixed to a micromanipulator.

The liquor obtained is observed in a monolayer preparation under a phase contrast microscope in a thermostat at the temperature of 38-39°C for the study of sanal in living conditions. [p71]

2. Form and size of sanal

The form and size of all sanal separated from the Bonghan duct of a rabbit are almost the same with one another when they are observed under a phase contrast microscope. When examined under a phase contrast microscope, the sanal separated from the Bonghan duct of man are almost the same as those taken out from the rabbit. And the forms of the sanal of mammals, birds, amphibians, fishes, etc. are also nearly the same. In plants too, the sanal similar to those in animals in form and size can be observed.

Sanal is usually spherical in shape but sometimes oval. An ordinary sanal is 1.2-1.5 microns in size, while the smallest one being 0.8 micron and the largest one, which is rarely found, is 2.4 microns.

Under the phase contrast microscope, each sanal has two parts—one is dark and the other is pale. The dark part, mostly located in the centre, is called Bonghan sanalosome, and the pale part surrounding it is called Bonghan sanaloplasm.

Sanal has a thin membrane, which is called sanal membrane. The sanalosome takes various forms—round, "ㅅ"-shaped, "ㅈ"-shaped, rod-shaped and star-shaped.

The sanalosome is positive in the Feulgen reaction and is well stained with basic dyes.

The sanaloplasm is poorly stained by basic dyes and shows no Feulgen reaction, but is stained red in the Brachet reaction.

The sanal membrane is thin but relatively durable, and its main chemical substance is lipoproteid.

The sanal membrane is easily destroyed by protein coagulants.

The detailed structure of sanal was studied under the electron microscope.

The sanalosome of various shapes is of high electron density, but sanaloplasm is comparatively of low density.

The sanal membrane is very dense and has a distinct contour.

Granules of relatively high electron density are seen in the sanaloplasm adjacent to the sanal membrane (Figure 72 on page 72).

Sanal make peculiar movements. When sanal in culture media are observed under the phase contrast microscope, they are found making constant rotating movements. The sanalosome also moves ceaselessly in the sanaloplasm.

The movements of sanal differ essentially from the Brownian movement of fine particles.

Sanal is sensitive to environment. Its movements are active at the temperature of 37-38°C and they slow down below 37°C. At [p72] temperatures above 56°C, the form of sanal changes and its movements stop. When acid, alkali and protein coagulants are added to the media, the sanaloplasm becomes destroyed, and its movements cease, too.

The movements of the sanal of plants are less active than those of the animal sanal.

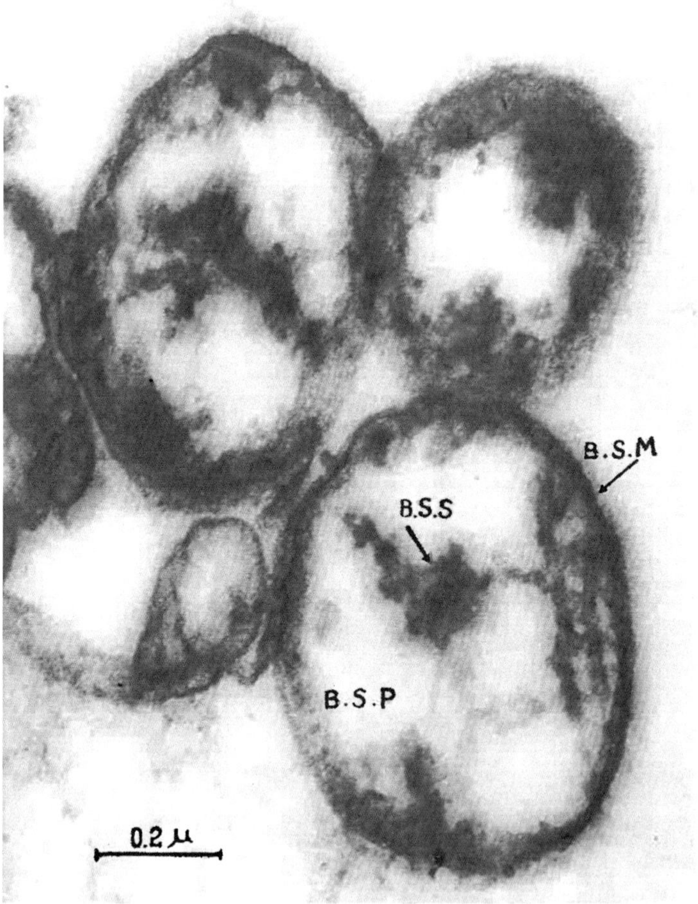

Figure 72. Electron micropragh of the Bonghan sanal (x117,000)

BSS — Bonghan sanalosome
BSP — Bonghan sanaloplasm
BSM — Bonghan sanal membrane

II. Biochemical study of sanal

Efforts were made to ascertain the chemical composition of sanal and the liquid menstruum of Bonghan liquor. The liquid menstruum, ie., the Bonghan liquor divested of sanal and other formed elements is called sanal fluid.

1. Main chemical composition of sanal

The sanal of the rabbit were analyzed. An isolated Bonghan duct was dissolved in the citric acid-sucrose solution and then sanal were suspended in the sucrose solution of different concentrations and were separated by density-gradient ultracentrifugation.

A) The contents of nucleic acids and protein in Bonghan sanal

The nucleic acids in sanal were estimated according to Schmidt-Thannhauser and Tsanev, and protein by the micro-Kjeldahl method respectively. Table 11 shows the contents of the nucleic acids and protein in a single Bonghan sanal.

As is seen in this Table, a sanal contains much nucleic acid, especially DNA, and a considerable amount of protein.

What merits particular attention is that the amount of DNA contained in one sanal is nearly equal to that contained in one chromosome. [p73]

Table 11. Contents of nucleic acids and protein in a Bonghan sanal (g)

DNA	RNA	Protein
$2.5 \cdot 10^{-13}$ ($2.0 \cdot 10^{-13} \sim 3.2 \cdot 10^{-13}$)	$1.2 \cdot 10^{-13}$ ($0.8 \cdot 10^{-13} \sim 1.6 \cdot 10^{-13}$)	$1.7 \cdot 10^{-12}$ ($1.2 \cdot 10^{-12} \sim 3.0 \cdot 10^{-12}$)

B) Molecular weight of DNA in sanal

The isolation of DNA from sanal was carried out by the chloroform method. The isolated nucleic acid contained 98.6 per cent of DNA and 0.8 per cent of RNA, and protein was scarcely recognizable.

The viscosity of DNA was determined with the Ostwald viscosimeter and then the molecular weight of the DNA was calculated by Spidkovsky's equation. The molecular weight of the DNA in sanal is estimated at 1.8×10^6 - 3.0×10^6.

C) Base composition of DNA and mononucleotide composition of RNA in sanal

We studied the base composition of DNA and the mononucleotide composition of RNA, which are the main components of sanal, by paper chromatography and paper electrophoresis.

One-dimensional descending chromatography was applied for the separation of the bases of DNA in the course of 15-40 hours; the solvent systems were n-butanol-water-caustic ammonia and methanol-hydrochloric acid-water.

The localization of spots on the developed paper was determined with the ultrachemiscope and each spot was estimated with the ultraviolet spectrophotometer. The following Table and Photos show the results of the analyses (Table 12 on page 74, and Figure 73 and Figure 74).

Table 12. Base composition of DNA (mol. %)

	Molar ration between bases (mol. %)
Guanine	21.85
Adenine	28.25
Cytosine + 5-Methylcytosine	21.30
Thymine	28.60

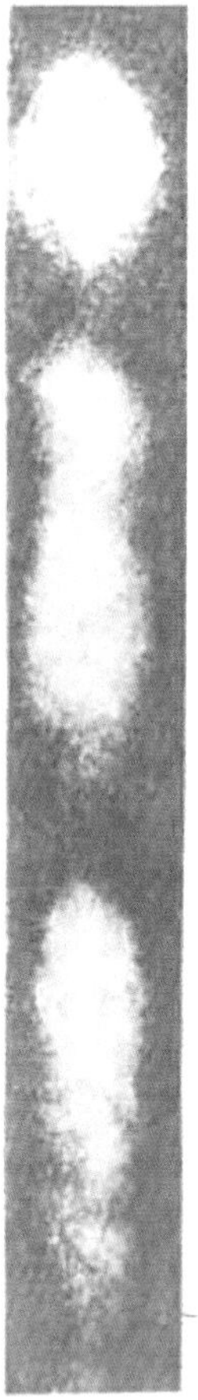

Figure 73. Paper chromatogram of bases of DNA in the Bonghan sanal

Solvent system:
methanol-hydrochloric acid-water

1. Guanine
2. Adenine
3. Cytosine
4. Thymine

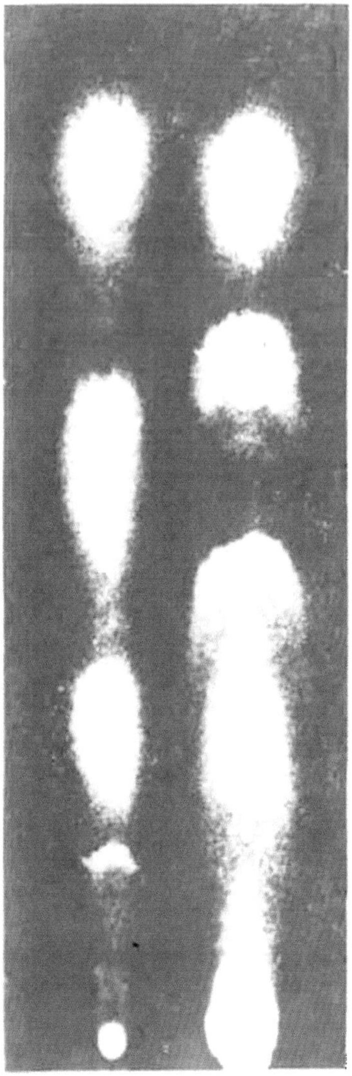

Figure 74. Paper chromatogram of bases of DNA in the Bonghan sanal

Solvent system: n-butanol-ammonia-water

a—standard; b—sanal

1. Guanine
2. Cytosine
3. 5-methyl-cytosine
4. Adenine
5. Thymine

The mononucleotide composition of RNA in sanal was analyzed by paper chromatography and paper electrophoresis. The solvent system used for paper chromatography was n-butanol-ammonia-water, and the buffer solution for electrophoresis was 0.5 mol acetic acid solution (27 v/cm, 2 mA/cm). [p74]

The results are presented in Table 13 and Figure 75 and Figure 76 on page 76.

Table 13. Mononucleotide composition of RNA (mol. %)

	Molar ratio between mononucleotides (mol. %)
Guanylic acid	29.58 – 33.49
Adenylic acid	18.50 – 21.09
Cytidylic acid	24.80 – 33.35
Uridylic acid	22.08 – 25.38

This base composition of DNA shows that DNA in sanal, just like that in the ordinary animal tissues, is of AT-type:

$$\left(\frac{\text{adenine} + \text{thymine}}{\text{guanine} + \text{cytosine} + \text{5-methylcytosine}} = \frac{28.25 + 28.60}{21.85 + 21.30} = 1.32 \right)$$

And the molar ratio of purine bases to pyrimidine bases is

$$\frac{21.85 + 28.25}{28.60 + 21.30} \approx 1$$

In the nucleotide composition of RNA of sanal the molar ratio of the sum total of guanylic and cytidylic acids to that of adenylic and uridylic acids is 1.34-1.50, while the molar ratio of purine bases to pyrimidine bases is 0.96-1.02.

D) Contents of mineral elements in sanal

The content of mineral elements in sanal was estimated by emission spectral analysis (semi-microanalysis) (wave length: 2,000-6,000 A.).

The results are given in Table 14.

As can be seen in Table 14, sanal contains a considerable amount of magnesium as well as iron, calcium, copper, manganese, zinc and cobalt.

Table 14. Contents of various mineral elements in dried sanal (%)

Copper	Magnesium	Iron	Manganese	Calcium	Zinc	Cobalt
$2\cdot10^{-3}$	$6\cdot10^{-1}$	$1\cdot10^{-1}$	$2\cdot10^{-3}$	$1\cdot10^{-1}$	$1\cdot10^{-4}$	$8\cdot10^{-6}$

Besides these, the analyses revealed the presence of lipids and carbohydrates in sanal.

After all, sanal is composed mainly of nucleic acids and proteins [p75] and it also contains carbohydrates, lipids and various inorganic substances.

Abundant proteins and important inorganic components in sanal are related with the presence of enzymes.

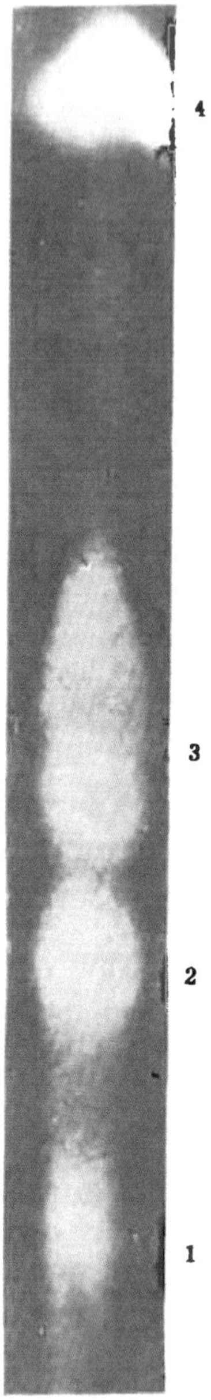

Figure 75. Paper chromatogram of RNA mononucleotides in the Bonghan sanal

Solvent system:
n-butanol-ammonia-water

1. Guanylic acid
2. Cytidylic acid
3. Uridylic acid
4. Adenylic acid

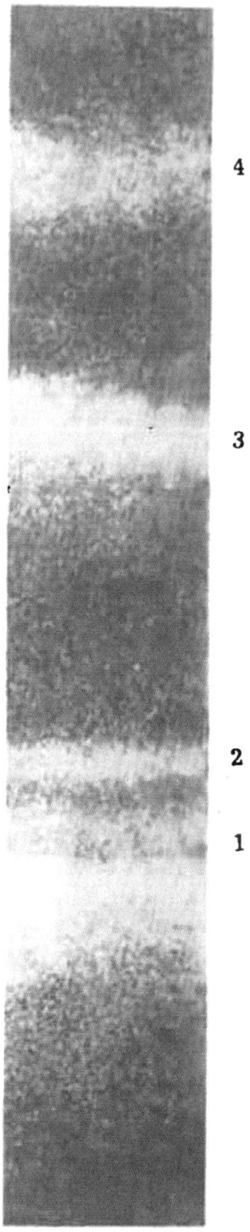

Figure 76. Electrophoregram of RNA mononucleotides in the Bonghan sanal

Buffer solution:
0.5 mol. acetic acid solution

1. Cytidylic acid
2. Adenylic acid
3. Guanylic acid
4. Uridylic acid

2. Main chemical composition of sanal fluid

After the removal of sanal and other formed elements by the high-speed centrifugation, we used the supernatant for analysis.

The total nitrogen and nonprotein nitrogen of sanal fluid was determined by the micro-Kjeldahl method and the determination of sugar was carried out after Hagedorn-Jensen, cholesterol according to Engelgardt, hyaluronic acid by ion exchange chromatography, free amino acids by high-voltage electrophoresis and paper chromatography, and free mononucleotides by ion exchange chromatography respectively (Table 15, Table 16, Table 18 on page 78; Figure 77 and Figure 78 on page 79). The findings are as follows: [p76]

Table 15. Contents of nitrogen, sugar, cholesterol and hyaluronic acid in sanal fluid (g%)

Total nitrogen	Nonprotein nitrogen	Reduced sugar	Cholesterol	Hyaluronic acid
1.50 – 2.55	0.07 – 0.11	0.08 – 0.10	0.032 – 0.048	0.14 – 0.18

Table 16. Contents of free amino acids in sanal fluid (mg%)

Amino acid	Content	Amino acid	Content
Leucine ± Isoleucine	8.47 ± 0.36	Asparagin	0.48 ± 0.06
Phenylalanine	1.89 ± 0.12	Lysine	3.11 ± 0.10
Valine + Methionine + Tryptophane	9.47 ± 0.11	Arginine	5.35 ± 0.13
Tyrosine	0.38 ± 0.02	Aspartic Acid	2.36 ± 0.21
Alanine	7.58 ± 0.38	Glutamine	0.41 ± 0.02
Glutamic acid	6.31 ± 0.29	Histidine	1.28 ± 0.09
Threonine	2.05 ± 0.23	Proline	—
Glycine + Serine	8.62 ± 0.61	Cystine	2.67 ± 0.14

As the Bonghan liquor is divided into sanal and sanal fluid, it is necessary to ascertain whether its DNA is contained in sanal or in sanal fluid. To this end we estimated DNA in sanal and sanal fluid according to Schmidt-Thannhauser. The ratio of contents of the DNA in sanal to that of sanal fluid is shown in Table 17.

Table 17. Ratio of DNA in sanal and in sanal fluid (%)

	Sanal	Sanal fluid
DNA	99.8	0.2

As is seen in the Table almost all DNA in the Bonghan liquor is contained in sanal.

Sanal fluid contains proteins, nonprotein nitrogen, reduced sugar, cholesterol and abundant hyaluronic acid, particularly various free amino acids and free mononucleotides. It is considered that these chemical components of sanal fluid circulating through the Bonghan ducts of the Kyungrak system are used in the metabolism of sanal when they grow into cells. [p77]

It is probable that sanal fluid is also of great importance in the metabolism of the tissue cells.

Table 18. Composition of free mononucleotides in sanal (mol/dl)

No.	Free mononucleotides	Contents
1	Cytosine monophosphate	0.25 ± 0.01
2	Nicotinadenine dinucleotide	21.60 ± 0.06
3	Adenosine monophosphate	9.20 ± 0.52
4	Inosine monophosphate	0.67 ± 0.12
5	Guanosine monophosphate	3.64 ± 0.52
6	Cytosine diphosphate	1.76 ± 0.02
7	Uridine monophosphate	2.14 ± 0.31
8	Inosine diphosphate	1.30 ± 0.09
9	Adenosine diphosphate ribose	2.34 ± 0.03
10	Adenosine diphosphate	4.89 ± 0.62
11	Cytosine triphosphate	12.29 ± 0.01
12	Uridine diphosphate	1.79 ± 0.04
13	Uridine diphosphate hexosamine	0.78 ± 0.04
14	Guanosine diphosphate	0.84 ± 0.36
15	Adenosine triphosphate	5.96 ± 0.06
16	Guanosine triphosphate	2.52 ± 0.12
17	Uridine triphosphate	2.10 ± 0.02

Figure 77. High voltage electrophoregram of free amino acids in the Bonghan sanal

Buffer solution:
pyridine solution (pH 6.5)

1. Aspartic acid
2. Glutamic acid
3. Histidine
4. Lysine
5. Arginine

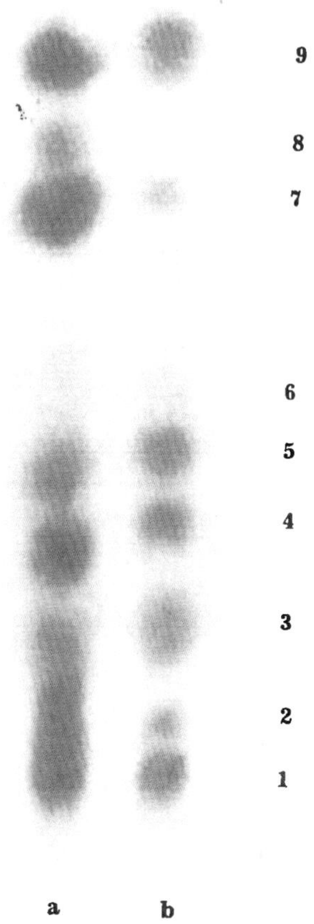

Figure 78. Paper chromatogram of free amino acids in the Bonghan sanal

a—standard; b—sanal fluid

1. Cystine
2. Asparagin
3. Glycine + Serine
4. Threonine
5. Alanine
6. Tyrosine
7. Valine + Methionine + Tryptophane
8. Phenyolalanine
9. Lecuine + Isoleucine

Chapter III. "Bonghan sanal-cell cycle"

In order to trace the processes of cell formation from a sanal, a single sanal was cultivated in vitro and the developments observed under the phase contrast microscope were cinematographed.

I. Culture method of sanal

For the culture of sanal in vitro, it is necessary, as in the case of ordinary tissue culture, to choose appropriate culture media and ensure the optimal conditions for the growth of sanal.

Through a series of experiments, we succeeded in preparing culture media suitable for the growth of sanal. The Other conditions like pH, osmotic pressure, temperature, viscosity, etc. required for their growth were so adjusted as to be fitted for ordinary cell culture.

A) Preparation of Culture Media

The following conditions are required in preparing culture media for the cultivation of sanal.

1) The composition of the media should be as similar as possible to that of Bonghan liquor because sanal grow in the Kyungrak system. Culture media with a composition resembling to that of Bonghan liquor should contain, first of all, mononucleotides, basis of nucleic acid, amino acids, carbohydrates, hyaluronic acid. etc.

2) Transparent liquid media are fitted for the observation of the movements and growth of sanal.

B) Cultivation of sanal

First of all, the sole sanal suspension should be prepared.

In order to get rid of alien elements which might be mixed up [p78] with sanal, sanal suspended in culture media are centrifugalized.

Sanal suspended in the sucrose solution are separated by density-gradient ultracentrifugation. Sanal are repeatedly washed with the culture media to get rid of sucrose, and a solely-separated sanal is cultivated either in culture flask or on slide-glass.

II. Cell formation from sanal

When a sanal is cultivated, it grows into a cell.

This process can be divided into two stages when we analyse its pictures taken through microcinematography.

A) The stage of proliferation

1) In the course of the movements of sanal, the sanalosome, changing itself into various forms, sends out a fine filiform process outside the sanal membrane.

2) Around the filiform process appears sanaloplasm and gradually grows in size. This is called daughter sanal. It grows nearly as large as the mother sanal.

3) The mother and daughter sanal form numerous daughter sanal in the same way. The sanal thus formed are not separable; because they are connected with each other by the filiform processes of sanalosomes.

4) Multiplied sanal present the appearance of a bunch of grapes.

B) The stage of fusion

1) The border line between sanal becomes indistinct and sanal unite each other. But the sanalosome still preserves its individuality.

2) A thin membrane is formed around the fused structure, which is called nucleus-like structure.

3) After the formation of the nucleus-like structure, homogeneous substance appears around it. This gradually grows and surrounds the nucleus-like structure.

4) The nucleus-like structure matures into a cell nucleus, while the homogeneous substance around it is transformed into cytoplasm. At the same time, the cell membrane is also formed (Figure 79). [p79]

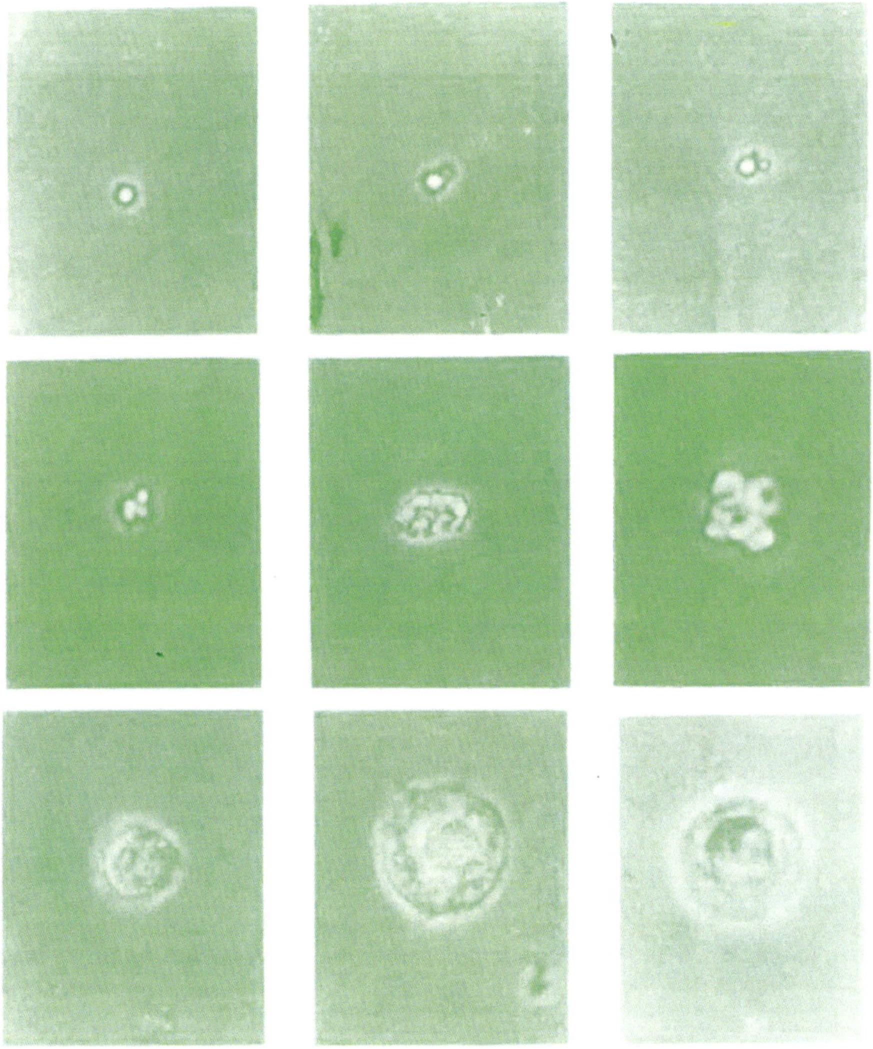

Figure 79. "Bonghan sanal-cell cycle" (Cell formation from sanal)

III. Sanalization of cell

Having confirmed the growth of Bonghan sanal into cells, we continued the research work to ascertain the fate of the cells thus formed and the origin of sanal.

It has been established that a cell again changes into sanal after some period of its existence, i.e., sanal has its own origin in the cell itself, not in anything else.

The process of the conversion of a cell into sanal is called the sanalization of a cell.

General forms of the processes are illustrated as follows:

After a definite period of time, dot-like structures begin to move in the nucleus of the cultured cell. These black dot-like substances gradually make active movements, grow larger, and form sanal.

Sanal which have been moving in the nuclei migrate into the cytoplasm, after the disappearance of the nuclear membrane.

Making active movements in the cytoplasm, sanal grow bigger.

With the active movements of sanal the cell membrane expands, and some time later it bursts to let the sanal out of the cell.

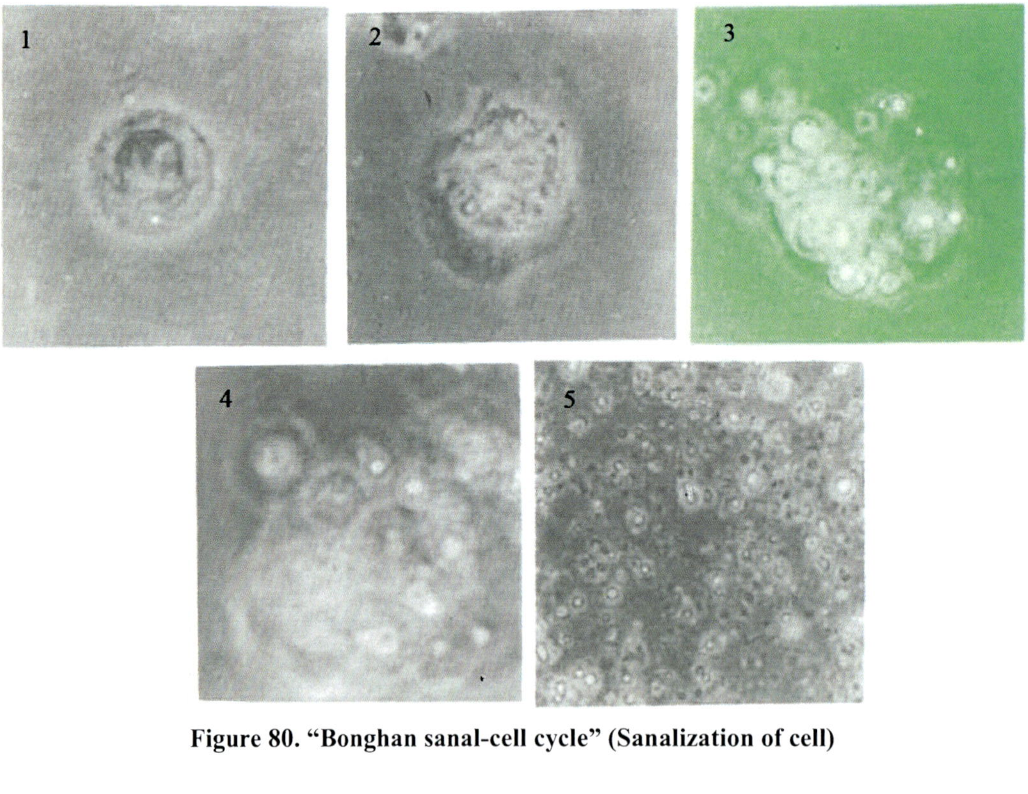

Figure 80. "Bonghan sanal-cell cycle" (Sanalization of cell)

Just before the rupture of the cell membrane, cytoplasmic substances are hardly to be seen in cytoplasm, but only sanal and small black granules are recognized.

With the rupture of a cell, these granules together with sanal burst out of the cell. The cell membrane preserves only its dim contour.

When a cell of normal tissues is separated from the living body the same process of sanalization is also to be recognized in it, and this process can be accelerated by various physico-chemical influences (Figure 80).

IV. "Bonghan sanal-cell cycle"

The growth of a sanal into a cell and the sanalization of a cell, both mentioned above, form a cyclic process.

Sanal, derived from a cell, again grow into cells. This process constitutes the "Bonghan sanal-cell cycle" (Figure 81).

Sanal collected from the Bonghan duct and Bonghan corpuscle can be changed into cells by cultivating them in vitro and vice versa.

Such a cycle is repeated also in the tissues of the living body. [p80]

Following are the experimental data about the "Bonghan sanal-cell cycle."

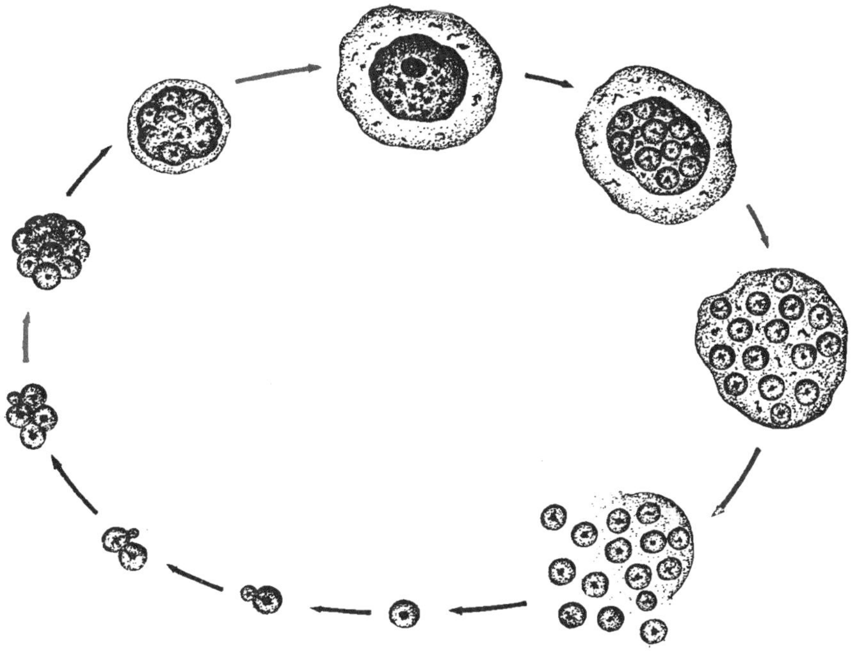

Figure 81. Diagram of "Bonghan sanal-cell cycle"

1) Sanal acquired from the internal Bonghan duct and internal Bonghan corpuscle of a rabbit liver were diluted with culture media, so as to fix a single sanal in the field of vision; and continued observations of it were made under the microscope. In 30 to 40 minutes' cultivation, the sanalosome protruded and then 40 minutes later it gave birth to a daughter sanal.

Sanal kept growing in number and entered the stage of fusion in 4-12 hours; they fused into a nucleus-like structure, either round or ovoid.

Around these structures a homogeneous, transparent plasm took shape and 72-120 hours after culture the cell membrane appeared to complete the formation of a cell.

The once formed cell was sanalized after about six to eight days (Figure 82 and Figure 83).

2) A sanal obtained through the sanalization of nerve cells of a rabbit brain begot two daughter sanal simultaneously by giving forth two sanalosomal filaments from sanalosome in 30 minutes' cultivation. Four to six hours later a sanal multiplied to 6 sanal, and 8 to 12 hours later to 12-13 sanal, assuming the shape of a long bunch of grapes. In 52 hours the sanal began to fuse to form a big, ovoid nucleus-like structure.

The cell thus formed takes the shape of a cross section of a vertebra, with clear cytoplasm and distinct membrane.

Out of the cell-body grow three projections, one of which becomes an axone.

3) When a sanal obtained through the sanalization of the proliferous discus of a chick embryo is cultivated, a cell is formed from the projections of the sanalosome in a comparatively shorter time. It takes 4-16 hours for a sanal to grow into a grape-bunch form, and the period of fusion is still shorter.

Generally, a sanal turns into a cell in 46-70 hours.

The sanal of the initial stage differ little in their size and shape, but the mature cells assume round, ellipsoidal and polygonal forms, and vary in size, too.

The forms and sizes of their nuclei were also different from each other.

When the cultivation of formed cells is continued, sanalization begins from bigger cells.

4) Sanal taken from fertilized eggs of a frog (Rana catesbiana) at the stage of 64 blastomeres were cultivated. [p81]

Sanal at the initial stage is 1.2-2.0 microns in size and the sanalosome looking slightly dark moves steadily.

Sanal grows very fast; in 12-22 hours it multiplies abundantly to take the form of a grape-bunch.

At that time the space between sanal is very wide and sanal are linked up with one another by the filaments of the sanalosomes. Twenty-two hours later, the fusion of sanal begins and it is completed in 28 hours.

After the fusion the nucleus-like structure appears usually ellipsoidal.

In 94 hours it grows into a cell with a large nucleus of distinct membrane.

Figure 82. Cells grown from sanal (x400)

5) In case of leukocytes, 90 minutes after culture, approximately four to five black granules are formed in the nucleus and in eight hours they increase in number. These granules come out of the nucleus, grow into sanal, moving in the cytoplasm, and the sanal come out of the cell. When a proper condition is provided from outside for the acceleration of this process, sanal burst out of the cell within one or two hours. These sanal grow into cells when cultivated.

6) A sanal was taken out of a young root cell of the sunflower right after the germination for the purpose of culture.

In four hours of culture a single daughter sanal took shape, and in 26 hours it multiplied to more than 10. Thirty hours after the culture the sanal began to fuse, and in 75 hours a cell formed. In the case of plants the process of the growth of sanal into cells is almost the same as to that of animals, but the peculiar feature here is that the mother sanal is always bigger than the daughter sanal.

Plant cells are also sanalized through prolonged cultivation.

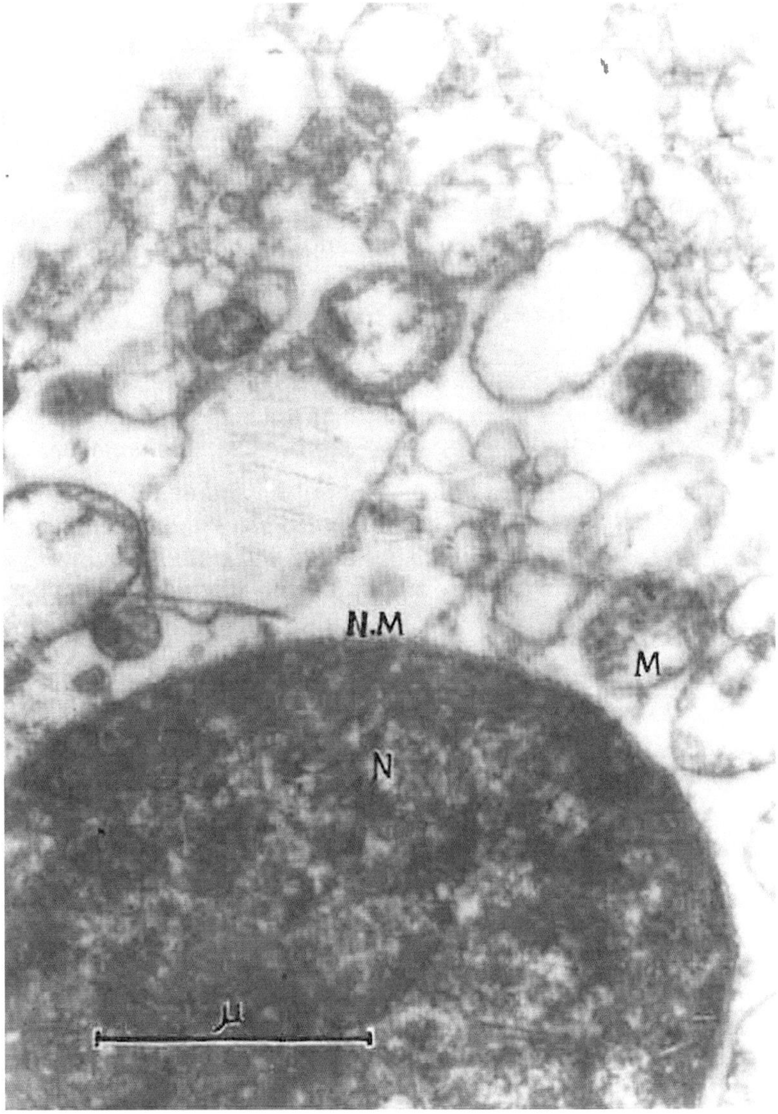

Figure 83. Electron micrograph of a cell grown from sanal (x37,000)
N—nucleus, NM—nuclear membrane, M—mitochondria

V. "Bonghan sanal-cell cycle" and biosynthesis

So far, morphological observations have been made on the process of the formation of a cell from a Bonghan sanal.

In order to clarify the biochemical dynamics of this process we analysed the content of nucleic acid, protein and amino acid in different stages of cell formation.

1) Materials

The sanal of the internal Bonghan duct of a rabbit were cultivated [p82] for 0, 24, 48, 72 and 144 hours respectively, and were examined under the phase contrast microscope, and biochemical analyses of them were carried out.

2) Findings in culture

It was observed under the phase contrast microscope that almost all the sanal measured 1.0-1.5 microns at the outset of culture and a lot of daughter sanal were formed from the mother sanal in 48 hours.

After 72 hours, the multiplied sanal were fused into many groups and 144 hours later many cells, either of the completed form or of being in the stage of formation of cytoplasm, were found in the culture media.

3) Nucleic acid and protein contents in different stages of culture

The isolation and measurement of nucleic acid in the materials were carried out according to Schmidt-Thannhauser and Tsanev. Table 19 shows the results of the analysis.

Table 19. Changes in contents of nucleic acids and protein nitrogen in cultivated sanal (r/%)

Time of culture (hr.)	DNA	RNA	Protein nitrogen
0	20.0 ± 5.1	33.3 ± 4.6	193.3 ± 7.5
24	85.9 ± 3.6	70.0 ± 4.9	1,773.3 ± 16.2
48	166.6 ± 3.1	163.3 ± 4.2	3,338.0 ± 21.6
72	329.6 ± 2.5	205.0 ± 4.0	4,115.0 ± 31.4
144	332.1 ± 3.2	302.1 ± 3.8	6,214.0 ± 62.0

In the course of the formation of a cell from a sanal, the contents of DNA increased 16 times (20.0:332.1), RNA: 9 times (33.3:302.1) and protein nitrogen 32 times (193.3:6,214.0).

As is shown in the above Table, the changes of each component according to the time of culture are diverse. It is illustrated in Figure 84. [p83]

As is shown in Figure 84, the content of DNA increased sharply from the beginning to 72 hours, and later very little. That is to say, during 24 hours ranging from 48 to 72 hours of cultivation the content of DNA doubled (166.6:329.6), whereas during 72 hours ranging from 72 to 144 hours it grew only a little bit (329.6:332.1).

When these results are compared with the morphological changes observed under the phase contrast microscope, it proves that the bio-synthesis of DNA takes place chiefly in the stage of proliferation of mother sanal into daughter sanal, and that the synthesis of DNA scarcely occurs while sanal are fused to form a nucleus and then cytoplasm. Contents of protein and RNA, however, show a steady increase after 72 hours of cultivation.

These data coincide with the morphological findings on the formation of cytoplasm and growth of the cell.

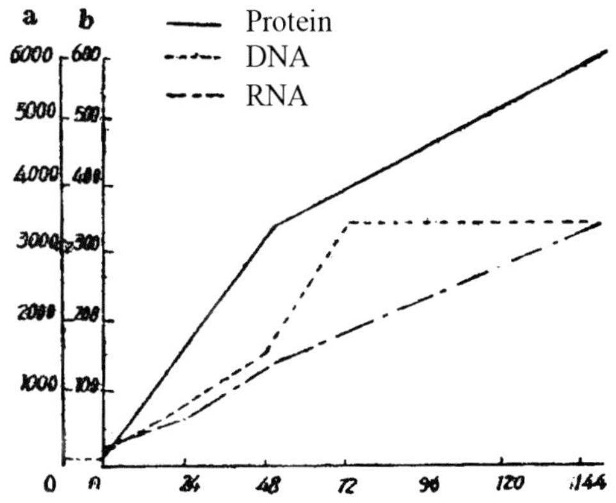

Figure 84. Changes of the contents of nucleic acid and protein according to the time of culture

a—Content of protein
b—Contents of DNA and RNA

4) Changes in the contents of protein amino acid according to the time of culture

Changes in the composition of protein amino acid- according to the time of culture were analyzed by paper chromatography and [p84] high-voltage electrophoresis. The solvent system for paper chromatography of amino acid was n-butanol-glacial acetic acid-water, and the buffer solution of pH 6.5 for high-voltage electrophoresis, was composed of pyridine-glacial acetic acid-water (supply of current 40 v/cm, 3 mA/cm).

The results are shown in

Table 20 and Figure 85 and Figure 86.

As is shown in Table 10, the contents of amino acid which was just traceable at the beginning of the culture increased rapidly according to the multiplication of sanal. Especially, the contents of arginine and glutamic acid, alanine, leucine, phenylalanine, aspartic acid, etc. showed a remarkable increase.

This indicates the energetic synthesis of protein de novo in the course of the multiplication of sanal and the formation of nuclei and cytoplasm. [p85]

Table 20. Contents of protein amino acid according to time of culture (mg %)

No.	Amino acid	Time of culture (hour)		
		0	48	144
1	Lysine	trace	0.20	0.60
2	Arginine	"	0.36	2.21
3	Histidine	"	0.11	0.33
4	Aspartic acid	"	0.34	1.36
5	Glutamic acid	"	0.34	1.56
6	Alanine	"	0.32	1.65
7	Tyrosine	—	trace	0.04
8	Glycine + Serine	trace	0.36	1.32
9	Cystine	—	0.20	0.50
10	Valine + Methionine + Tryptophane	trace	0.40	2.20
11	Phenylalanine	"	0.25	1.50
12	Leucine + Isoleucine	"	0.50	2.01
13	Proline	—	trace	0.72
14	Threonine	trace	0.06	0.24

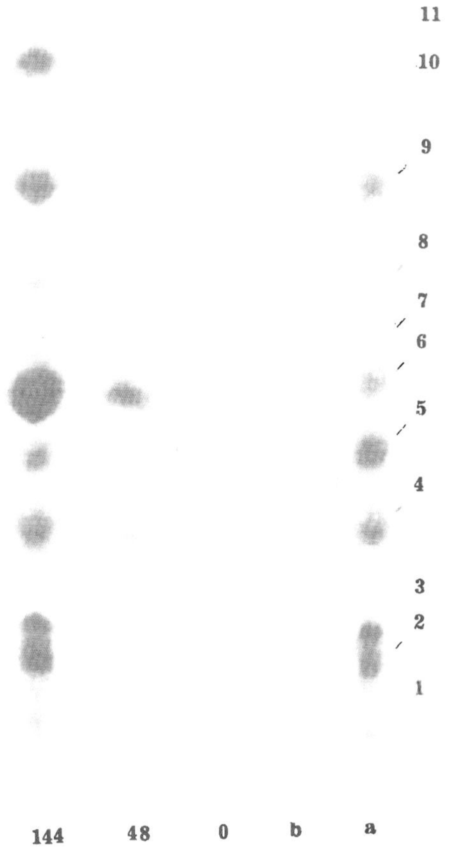

Figure 85. Paper chromatogram of protein amino acid

a—Standard
b—Culture media
0—At the outset of culture
48—Cultivated for 48 hours
144—Cultivated for 144 hours

Solvent system: n-butanol-glacial acetic acid-water

1. Cystine
2. Glycine + Serine
3. Threonine
4. Alanine
5. Proline
6. Tyrosine
7. Methionine + Valine + Tryptophane
8. Phenylalanine
9. Leucine + Isoleucine

Figure 86. High voltage paper electrophoregram of protein amino acid

0—At the outset of culture
48—Cultivated for 48 hours
144—Cultivated for 144 hours

Buffer solution: pyridine solution (pH 6.5)

1. Aspartic acid
2. Glutamic acid
3. Histidine
4. Lysine
5. Arginine

Chapter IV. Sanal and cell division

Having confirmed that the formation of cells through the "Bonghan sanal-cell cycle" exists objectively in the organism, we examined the well-known phenomena of cell division from a new point of view.

Studies of cell division were done in the living specimen under the phase contrast microscope and comparisons were made with histological preparations.

In the inter-phase of cell division individual sanal in the nucleus are in a fused state and are scarcely recognizable. In the histological preparations of this phase only chromatin particles and nucleoli are to be seen. When observed under the phase contrast microscope, punctate structures appear in the nucleus and begin to move at the outset of the cell division.

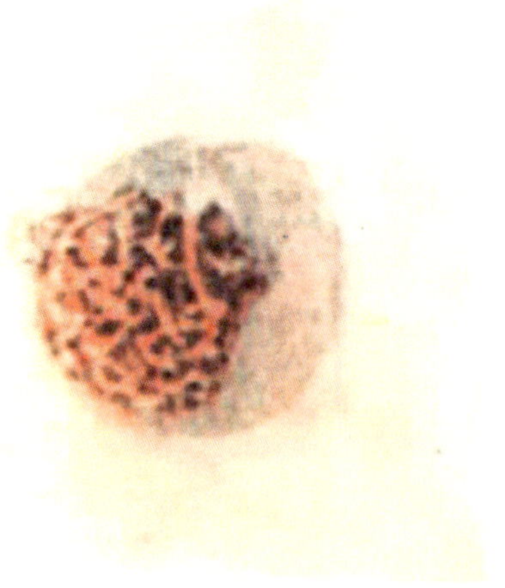

Figure 87. Initial stage of the cell division (Sanalized nucleus) (x1,000)

As time passes, these punctate structures grow and become brilliant, invigorating their motion (Figure 87). Then, nuclear membrane disappears, letting them go into the cytoplasm. These punctate structures are nothing but sanal. If a section of this period is fixed and stained with Giemsa, the chromatin appears purple (Figure 88). The punctiform or rod-shaped, deeply-stained granules are sanalosomes.

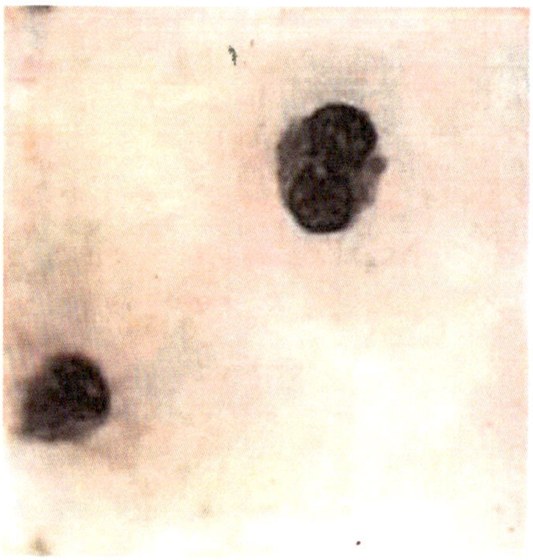

Figure 88. Cell division (Sanal came our of the nucleus into the cytoplasm) (x1,000)

The sanal which invaded into the cytoplasm grow in size and show more brisk motion.

The cell gradually takes an ellipsoidal shape, while the sanal continue active motions. At this time most of the sanal in cytoplasm are seen separately in histological preparations.

The sanal gather in the centre of the cell and then migrate towards its both poles.

The migrated groups of sanal on each pole are fused and then form nucleus-like structures (Figure 89).

At this time the nuclear membrane as well as nucleolus are also formed. Simultaneously the elongated cell is constricted in the middle part and a line appears leading to the division of cytoplasm into two.

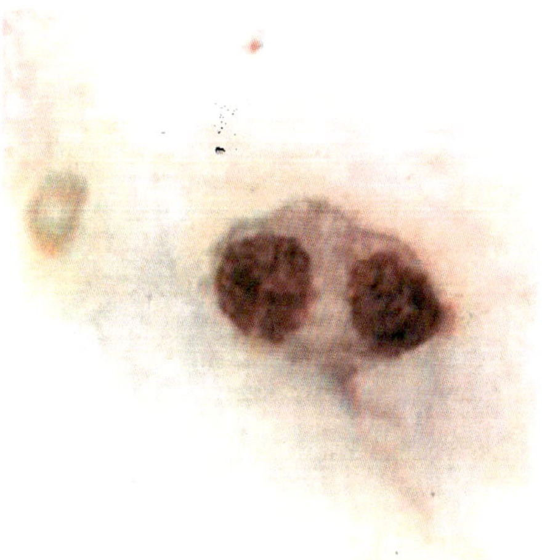

Figure 89. Cell division (Sanal appeared in the cytoplasm are grouped and form two nuclei) (x1,000)

In histological preparations, it is observed that nuclei are formed, [p86] the cell membranes become distinct and the cytoplasm contracts in the middle part and then divided.

Thus, two daughter cells are formed (Figure 90).

When this whole process is reviewed it can be stated that the cell division is a mode of cell multiplication by means of separation, migration, and fusion in groups of sanal which are born through the preceding sanalization of the cell (Figure 91 on page 93).

Experimental case 1: Division of the corneal epithelial cell of a tadpole (R. catesbiana).

A living specimen of separated corneal epithelium was observed under the phase contrast microscope.

In the first stage, punctate structures appear gradually in the nucleus. With the lapse of time, they grow bigger and brighter and begin to move.

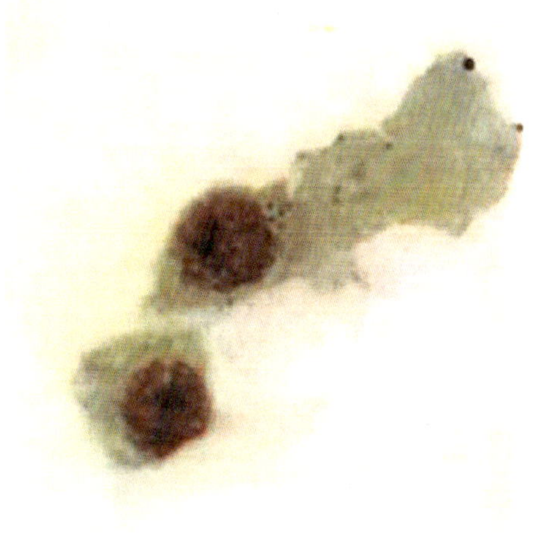

Figure 90. Cell division (Nuclei are completed and cytoplasm is divided into two daughter cells) (x1,000)

Then the nuclear membrane disappears, letting the sanal go into the cytoplasm.

The sanal which have been moving in the cytoplasm migrate towards both poles and are fused.

Around the fused structures appear membranes, bringing nuclei into being. At this time the middle part of the cytoplasm is constricted and gradually divided into two.

Experimental case 2: Division of the epidermal cell of a chick embryo.

An epidermal cell was separated from the chick embryo on the eighth day of incubation and its living specimen was observed.

Black spots appear in the nucleus which looked homogeneous at first, and growing in size, they look bright. The newly formed sanal begin to move.

The nuclear membrane disappears and the sanal go into the cytoplasm.

In the cytoplasm the sanal migrate to the poles, then they fuse to form nuclei.

With the formation of the nuclei, the cytoplasm also gradually splits and two daughter cells are formed.

The whole process takes place within 180 minutes.

Experimental case 3: Cell division of the proliferous discus of a chick embryo.

The cell division of the proliferous discus occurs within a short time.

The granules which appear as small dots at first, grow gradually into sanal and begin active movement and split towards the poles.

The cytoplasm gets constricted in the middle part, where a black line appears, finally dividing cytoplasm. [p87]

The sanal at both poles gradually form nuclei. It takes 70 minutes to complete this process.

These findings suggest that the movements of sanal have something in common with those of the chromosome. That is, the behavior of the sanalosome in the course of cell division under the phase contrast microscope is the same to the well-known behavior of the chromosome.

When the cell is fixed and stained just before the migration of the newly formed sanal towards the poles of the cell, and observed under the microscope, the sanalosomes, assuming rod, thread-like or dot shapes, bear the same appearance to what is known as the chromosome.

The number of sanal at the time of cell division is similar to that of chromosome.

As mentioned above, the sanalosome is basophile and shows positive Feulgen reaction, and the content of DNA is similar to that of the chromosome.

In a nutshell, it is regarded that the chromosomes appearing at the time of cell division are nothing but sanalosomes, and that the cell division is essentially a specific form of the movements of sanal.

Cell division can be regarded as the whole process of the "Bonghan sanal-cell cycle" taking place in a cell. That is, the cell division can be called intracellular "Bonghan sanal-cell cycle," a specific form of the "Bonghan sanal-cell cycle."

This process, however, is united with the extracellular "Bonghan sanal-cell cycle" (Figure 92 on page 93).

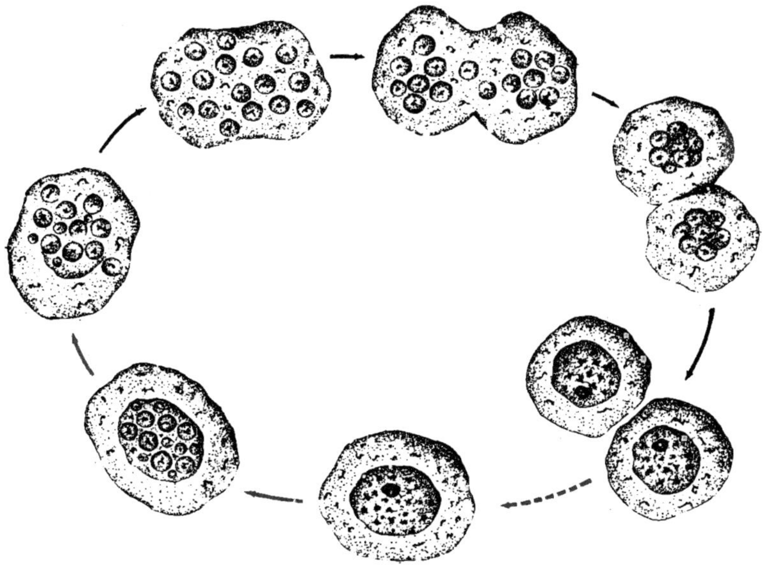

Figure 91. Diagram of “Bonghan sanal-cell cycle” (intracellular)

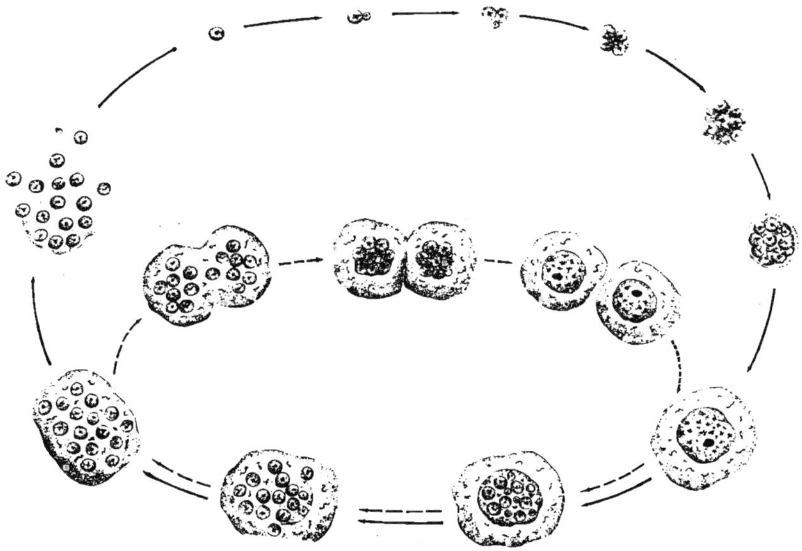

Figure 92. Diagram of "Bonghan sanal-cell cycle" (intracellular and extracellular)

Chapter V. Sanal and cell

The cell theory holds that the cell is the unitary morphological and functional unit of the organism and that cells are formed only from cells through cell division.

Our experimental results, however, demand a re-examination of this aspect.

Hence there arises the necessity of studying the correlation between sanal and the cell. Two ways of interpretation might be possible as to the process of the formation of a nucleus through the fusion of sanal. [p88]

One is that each sanal, when fusing, preserves its individuality, while the border between sanal becomes indistinct simply because of physico-chemical factors, and then the sanal regains its proper appearance with the change of the physico-chemical conditions. The other is that sanal loses its individuality, while forming a nucleus, and then recovers it in the course of sanalization.

The former interpretation is supported by the fact that a certain physical or physico-chemical influence alone can make a resting nucleus exhibit its clear sanal structure and thus sanalize in a short time.

Nevertheless, it should be considered that sanal undergoes some changes in the whole course of fusion and dissociation. Differences are noted between sanal inside the nucleus and those outside the cell.

A cell is not a simple mechanical congregation of sanal. Careful study of the process of sanalization of a cell revealed that black dots (equivalent to sanalosomes), while moving in the nucleus, absorb something of the karyoplasm, then come out of the nucleus in the cytoplasm and get substances from the cytoplasm, and thus the black dots that are sanal acquire their whole features.

Sanal in the cell nucleus, therefore, differ from those outside the cell.

A sanal has two stages: the stage in a resting nucleus and the stage outside the cell. The stage of fusion of sanal and the stage of sanalization of the cell are the transitional stages between these two.

Sanal is not in stationary condition, but is in constant motion. In other words, it repeats a cyclic movement. It is clear that this movement is based on the qualitative changes of sanal.

In the course of cell division, sanal takes various forms at each stage, and when the cell division is complete, sanal returns to its original state.

What has hitherto been called chromosome in cell division is nothing but the sanalosome, and the so-called behaviour of the chromosome is the very behaviour of sanal in cytoplasm.

This leads to the conclusion that the cell is a specific stage in the cyclic movement of sanal. [p89]

Chapter VI. "Bonghan sanal-cell cycle" and the role of the Kyungrak system

Studies on the process of the "Bonghan sanal-cell cycle" have so far been made mainly under the conditions of culture in vitro.

Based on these data, further study has been made to ascertain this "Bonghan sanal-cell cycle" in the living body, the process which is regarded as the basic form of self-renovation in the organism.

In order to demonstrate that the "Bonghan sanal-cell cycle" takes place in the living body, the following questions should be answered:

1) Does sanalization occur in every tissue cell of the living body?

2) If sanalization does occur in the tissue cells, do sanal move through the circulation route of the Bonghan liquor?

3) Do sanal mature in that route?

4) Do sanal, thus matured, again grow into cells?

Following studies have been made to solve these questions.

I. Distribution of sanal

If the sanal formed in the tissue cells grow while flowing with Bonghan liquor in the Kyungrak system, sanal at various stages of maturity should be found only in the Kyungrak system. To prove this, the distribution of sanal was studied in the living body.

In the organism sanal exist only in the Kyungrak system and they are scarcely found in blood, lymph and tissue fluid. In the Kyungrak system sanal are found in all the Bonghan ducts and corpuscles. Moreover, sanal in different stages of maturity are observed in the ducts and corpuscles. [p90]

1. In the Bonghan duct

A) In the intravascular Bonghan duct sanal of the initial stage measuring 1.2-1.4 microns are predominant, and those in different stages of growth are also to be seen.

There is difference between the sanal of the Bonghan duct in the artery and those in the vein.

Two kinds of sanal are recognized in the internal Bonghan duct of the artery of a rabbit; one is 1.5 microns in size with pale sanaloplasm, and the other is 0.8-1.0 micron in size with somewhat dark sanaloplasm.

The sanal within the Bonghan duct in the caudal vena cava of a rabbit measures 1.0-1.5 microns, its plasm being pale. Besides these, small sanal of about 0.3 micron and large ones of some 2.0 microns are also found.

B) The size of sanal in the external Bonghan ducts does not differ from the size of those in the internal Bonghan ducts; in the former there are many bigger sanal measuring some 1.5-2.0 microns.

C) The intra-external Bonghan ducts contain sanal of 1.0-1.8 microns and the refractivity of the sanalosomes is rather low.

2. In the Bonghan corpuscle

Particularly numerous are the multiplied sanal in the Bonghan corpuscle.

A) The superficial Bonghan corpuscle

The size of the sanal in the superficial Bonghan corpuscle of a rabbit reaches 1.4-1.8 microns and the sanaloplasm looks rather pale.

The sanalosomes are relatively big, and they have various forms such as punctate, "ᄉ"-form, "ᄌ"-form and rod-shape. The sanal of light plasm are found with two-three or more daughter sanal.

In the frog, the sanal in the superficial Bonghan corpuscle have the same forms and sizes as those of the rabbit, but the sanalosomes are bigger than those of the latter.

Some sanal in the superficial Bonghan corpuscle of man are oval measuring 1.5 microns in size, and the forms of the sanalosomes are diverse.

B) The intra-external Bonghan corpuscle

The sanal in the intra-external Bonghan corpuscle have the same appearances as those in the ducts linked to it, but the developed sanal [p91] are found more abundantly than in the former.

The fact that sanal exist only in the Kyungrak System means that they can grow only in this system.

Bonghan liquor contains an abundance of various substances necessary for the growth of sanal, that is, mononucleotides, bases of nucleic acid, and free amino acids. Besides reduced sugar and lipids, it also contains hormones, including adrenocortical and adrenomedullary hormones, sex hormones as well as a lot of hyaluronic acid.

A sanal can not be cultivated in blood serum, lymph and tissue fluid.

II. Circulation of sanal

It is considered that sanal found only in Bonghan liquor should doubtlessly move into the tissue cells of every organ through the circulating routes of the Bonghan liquor, and that sanal should grow in the Bonghan liquor which ensures conditions for their growth.

Proceeding from the necessity of verifying this fact, P32-tagged sanal were used and traced by microautoradiography.

Sanal were taken out of the superficial Bonghan corpuscle, internal Bonghan duct and tissue cells. Suspension of sanal, containing 50μC of $Na_2\ HP^{32}\ O_4$ per ml was cultivated for a definite period of time to label sanal.

Labelled sanal were isolated by centrifugation, the supernatant containing unutilized phosphate being discarded. Labelled sanal were repeatedly washed until the radioactivity of the supernatant dropped to that at a natural level.

Tagged sanal were injected into different parts of the circulating route of Bonghan liquor.

Experiments were repeated to ascertain the route of sanal after sanalization in the tissue cells.

1. Injection of P32-tagged Sanal

Tagged sanal were injected into the internal Bonghan duct of organs. And radioautography was applied to the circulation course of Bonghan liquor and to the different tissues of internal organs, where the injected sanal were supposed to be circulating, in 30 minutes and in 3, 6, 12, 24, 36 and 48 hours after the injection.

Following are some examples: [p92]

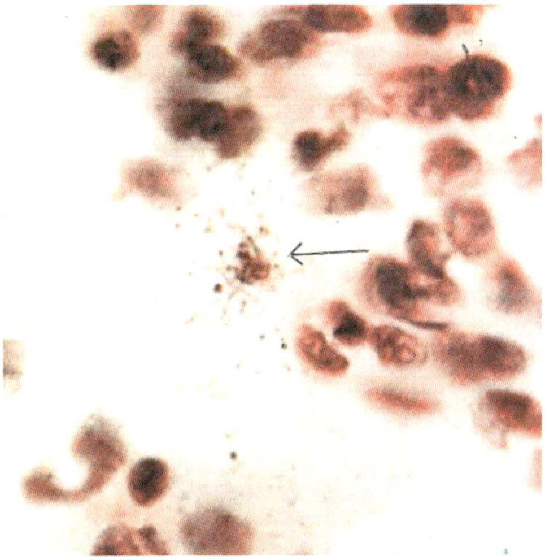

Figure 93. Microautoradiogram of the lung tissue (Nucleus-like structures labelled after 30 mins in the liver when P32-tagged Bonghan sanal were injected into the internal Bonghan duct)

(1) Focussed on the file of the nuclear emulsion (x1,000)

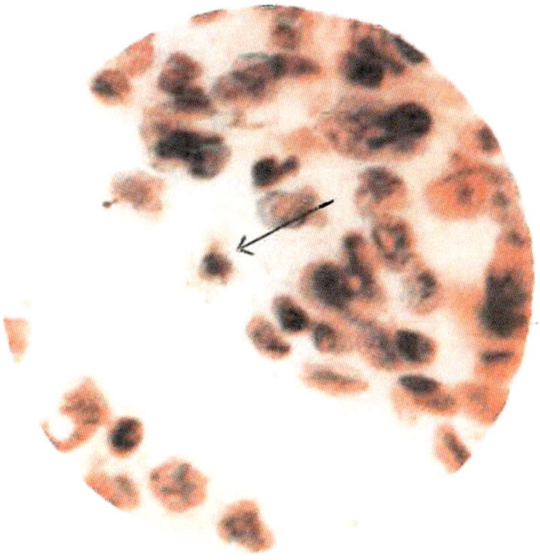

(2) Focussed on the section (x1,000)

A) In the lung

Thirty minutes after the injection, one or two to three labelled nucleus-like structures of 3-4 microns in size, round or oval, deep basophile, were observed separately, or clustered among the alveolar epithelial cells (Figure 93).

As a rule, sanal do not take the form of a cell up to 12 hours after the injection, but they are multiplied and grown. In the alveolar epithelial cells nucleus-like structures, round and basophile, measuring 5-6 microns and having no cytoplasm, are seen labelled in 24 hours after the injection of labelled sanal.

In 48 hours after the injection, alveolar epithelial cells nearly matured are found. They are similar to the surrounding alveolar epithelial cells; their cytoplasm is comparatively scanty and their nuclei are deeply stained with basic dyes (Figure 94 on page 98).

At this moment the labelled nucleus-like structures at different stages can be recognized.

B) In the liver

Data similar to those in the above case were obtained; 30 minutes later the labelled nucleus-like structures, separate or grouped by twos and threes were to be seen between liver cells and between cell cords. They were approximately 2-3 microns in size, round or ellipsoidal, and deep basophile (Figure 95 on page 98, and Figure 96 on page 99).

Twenty-four to thirty-six hours after the injection, tagged round nucleus-like structures are to be seen. By that time cytoplasm is hardly recognized. In 48 hours after the injection, labelled liver cells can be seen among the proper liver cells; the nuclei of these cells are somewhat easily stainable and are similar to those of the surrounding cells in size, and the cytoplasm is scanty and faintly stained.

These facts suggest that the labelled sanal injected into the Kyungrak system multiply and form cells with the lapse of time.

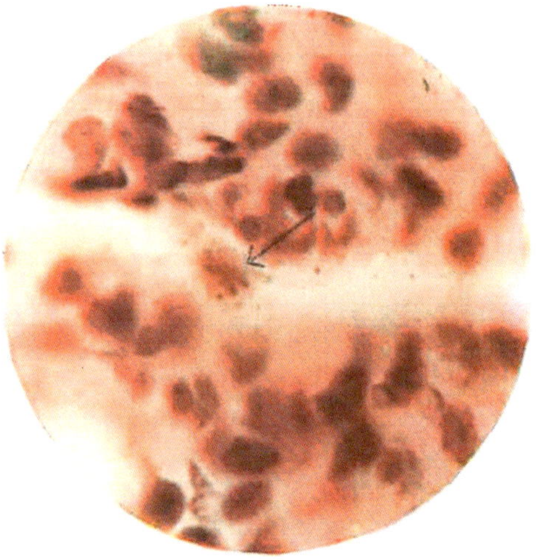

Figure 94. Microautoradiogram of the lung tissue (Alveolar epithelial cells labelled after 48 hours when P32-tagged Bonghan sanal were injected into the internal Bonghan duct)

(1) Focussed on the film of the nuclear emulsion (x1,000)

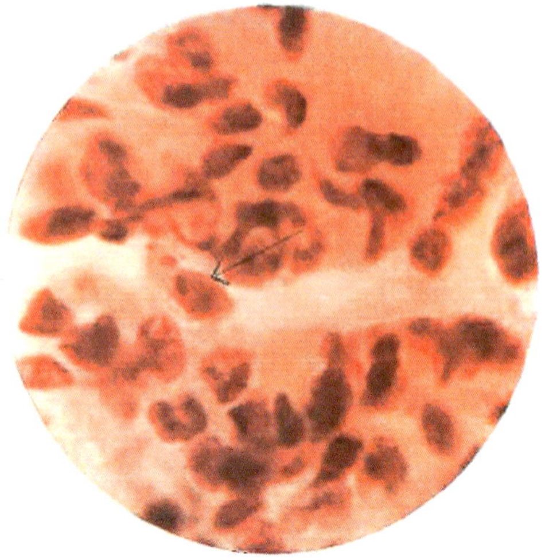

(2) Focussed on the section (x1,000)

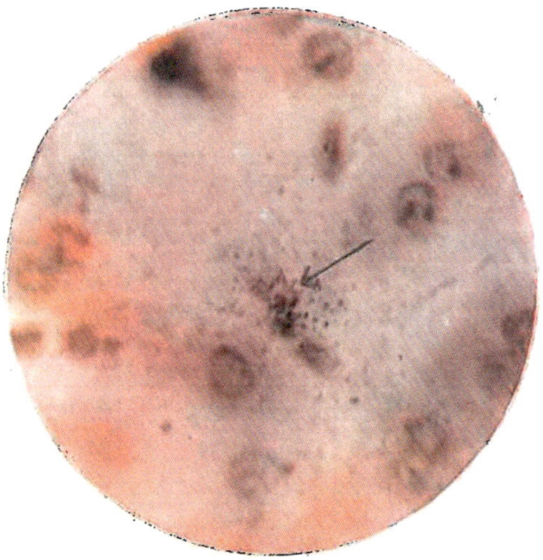

Figure 95. Microautoradiogram of the liver tissue (Nucleus-like structures labelled after 30 minutes in the liver when P32-tagged Bonghan sanal were injected into the internal Bonghan duct)

(1) Focussed on the film of the nuclear emulsion (x1,000)

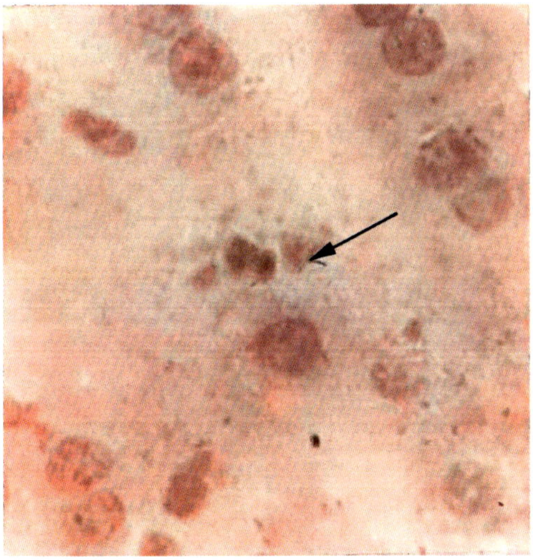

(2) Focussed on the section (x1,000)

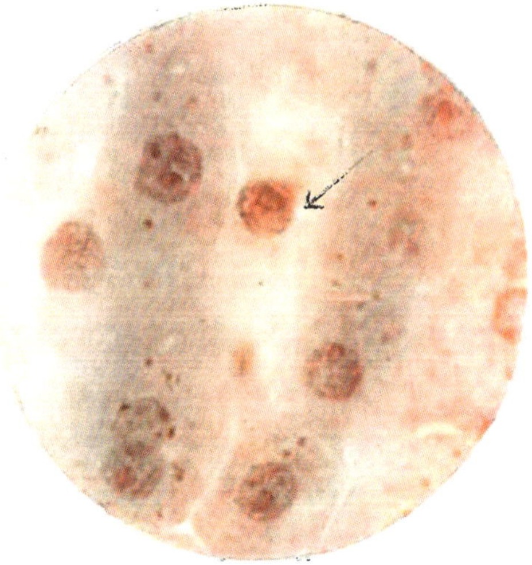

(2) Focussed on the section (x1,000)

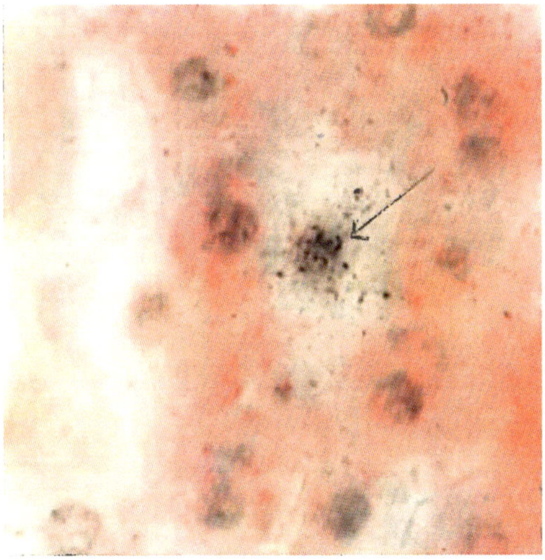

Figure 96. Microautoradiogram of the liver tissue (Liver cells labelled after 48 hours when P32-tagged Bonghan sanal were injected into the internal Bonghan duct)
(1) Focussed on the film of the nuclear emulsion (x1,000)

C) In the kidney

Three hours after the injection, oval, basophile nucleus-like structures measuring 3-4 microns can be observed between the epithelial cells of straight uriniferous tubules, and between those of the convoluted uriniferous tubules (Figure 97).

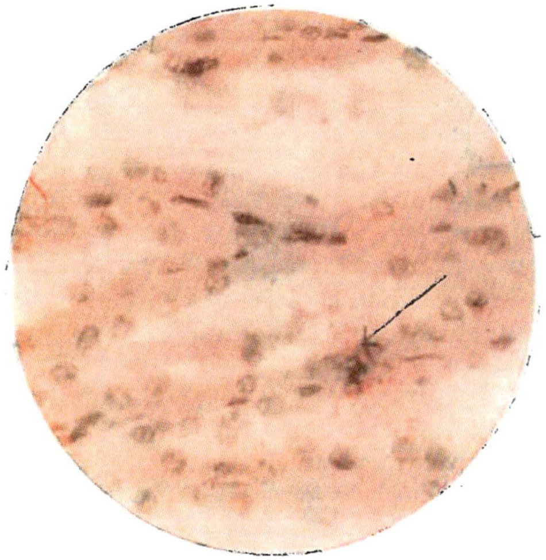

Figure 97. Microautoradiogram of the kidney tissue (Nucleus-like structures labelled after 3 hours in the kidney when P32-tagged Bonghan sanal were injected into the internal Bonghan duct) (x400)

New labelled cells appear between the epithelial cells of uriniferous tubules in 48 hours. These findings mean that sanal multiply and form new cells in the kidney as well. [p93]

D) In the ovary, suprarenal body and other organs the same findings were recorded (Figure 98, page 100)

These experimental data were fully confirmed by control experiments.

When the suspension containing the same number of labelled sanal as in the foregoing experiments was injected into blood vessels, the results obtained were not similar to those mentioned above.

The results obtained are summarized as follows:

1) Sanal formed in the internal organs are considered to migrate into the superficial Bonghan corpuscles, and as time passes, again return to the internal organs.

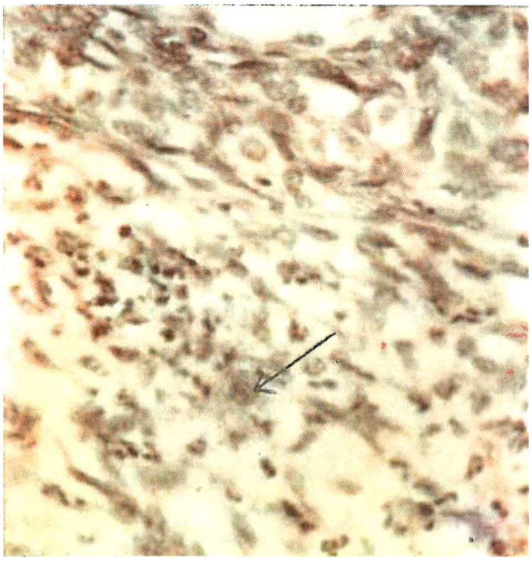

Figure 98. Microautoradiogram of the ovary tissue (Nucleus-like structures labelled when P32-tagged Bonghan sanal were injected into the internal Bonghan duct) (x400)

2) Sanal injected into the superficial Bonghan corpuscle grow large and become nucleus-like structures on their way to different internal organs through Bonghan ducts, and they again move through intraorganic Bonghan ducts and grow into cells in the internal organs.

And sanal injected into the superficial Bonghan corpuscle are conveyed to the external, intra-external and internal Bonghan corpuscles.

3) Sanal of the superficial Bonghan corpuscle, when injected into the Bonghan duct, grow into cells in the internal organs.

The above-mentioned results imply that sanal formed in the tissue cells are carried to the superficial Bonghan corpuscles through Bonghan ducts, then to the profund Bonghan corpuscles and that they form tissue cells, passing through different intraorganic corpuscles.

To prove this more clearly, the following experiments were conducted.

2. Culture of sanal picked from superficial Bonghan corpuscle

As sanal formed in the tissue cells of different organs pass through the definite superficial Bonghan corpuscles, various cells would be obtained if sanal are taken from the corpuscles and cultivated.

The centuries-old experiences in acupuncture show that superficial Bonghan corpuscles in different regions have specific connections with relevant internal organs.

If so, different cells would be formed from sanal taken from different corpuscles. Taking the clinical findings into consideration, we cultivated on 344 occasions the sanal taken from the superficial Bonghan corpuscles in 79 regions of the human body. As had been expected, different cells were formed in accordance with the loci of those superficial Bonghan corpuscles. This means that the sanal formed in the tissue cells [p94] of different organs pass through the superficial Bonghan corpuscles linked with the internal organs.

We also studied what kind of influence is exerted upon sanal in the superficial Bonghan corpuscle.

The histological findings that the network of Bonghan ductules distributed in the outer layer of the superficial Bonghan corpuscle containing abundant sanal is connected with epidermis, and the data obtained through the stain painting and the stain injecting experiments confirm that sanal circulate through the superficial corpuscle and its upper parts.

Surmising that photochemical influence might be one of the important ones exerted on sanal in the superficial Bonghan corpuscle, we tried to prove this.

When sanal are cultivated in a dark chamber, less sanal grow into cells.

For instance, sanal taken from liver cells were cultivated, some in a dark chamber, others in normal light, and the results were compared.

Under normal light 104 cells were formed in 96 hours, whereas in the dark chamber only 32 were formed during the time.

When sanal taken from the spleen were cultivated in the same way, 69 cells were formed in 96 hours under normal conditions, whereas in the dark chamber the multiplication of sanal stopped utterly in 72 hours and no more cells were formed thereafter.

Similar data were obtained in other experiments. The growth of several sanal into cells in a dark chamber is explained by the fact that a few sanal already influenced by light in the superficial Bonghan corpuscle before the separation were mixed among the cultivated sanal.

III. "Bonghan sanal-cell cycle" in normal tissues

To demonstrate the process of "Bonghan sanal-cell cycle" in the organism, it was necessary to ascertain whether sanal grow into cells and cells are sanalized in the normal tissue cells.

The above-mentioned data have confirmed that the sanal formed in the tissue cells mature and grow into cells while migrating through the circulation route of Bonghan liquor. However, it is not yet known how mature sanal grow into cells in tissues and cells turn into sanal in the organism.

To demonstrate this, preparations of normal tissue were examined [p95] from a new point of view; and at the same time, frozen sections of vital tissue were made and immersed in culture media and studied under the phase contrast microscope for many hours in living conditions and then they were fixed and stained for observation.

By the latter method, each stage of the sanalization of tissue cells was clearly to be seen in vital preparations.

The normal liver tissues of the rabbit and pig were used as experimental materials, and histological preparations of hematoxylin-eosin stain were examined.

1. Process of sanalization

Liver cells are generally polygonal and bordered clearly; their cytoplasm is rather deeply stainable; round nuclei are usually situated at the centre of the cell body; and each nucleus has clearly discernible nucleoli, chromatin granules and the nuclear membrane, etc.

In some cells, the cell membrane appears broken and the cytoplasm scattered, being poorly stainable. The nuclei of such cells contain granular chromatins, the nuclear membranes are thin and parts of them bulge out (Figure 99 on page 102).

There are also cells which, similar as they are to the abovementioned cells morphologically, have nuclear membranes bulging and ruptured in part and some chromatin granules lying in the cytoplasm. Among these cells with ruptured nuclear membranes there are various kinds of cells including those much of whose chromatin has migrated out of the nuclei or only a few of whose chromatin granules have migrated out (Figure 100).

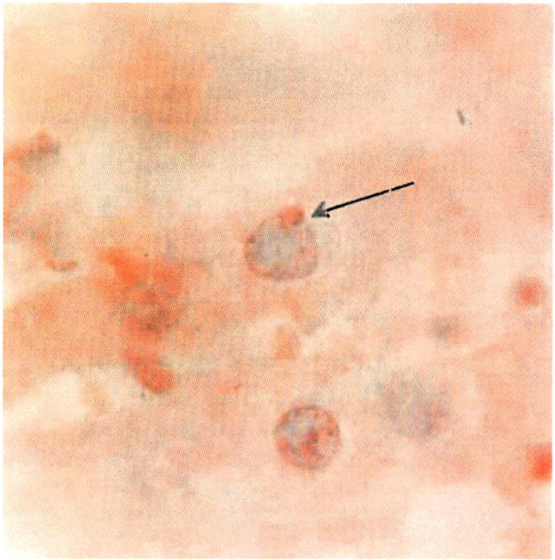

Figure 99. Nucleus at the outset of sanalization (x1,000)

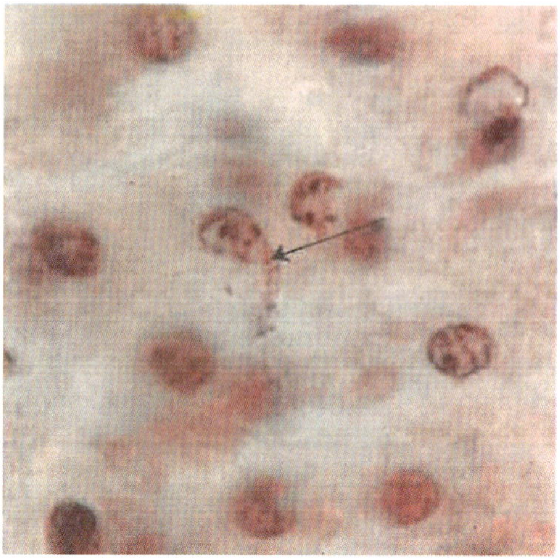

Figure 100. Nucleus in the course of sanalization (x1,000)

In some cells it is observed that the cytoplasm is more obscure and part of the deformed nuclear membrane is found, basophile granules being lined obliquely around it. The more granules are outside the nucleus, the more severely destroyed the cell is. And there are cells in which the cytoplasm is thoroughly destroyed, and only the residue of the nuclear membrane is recognized with difficulty and no chromatin is found in it. Such cells whose cell membranes are ruptured have communication with the sinusoid.

In the sinusoid there are chromatin granules lying in a line and seeming to be covered with very thin membranes (Figure 101).

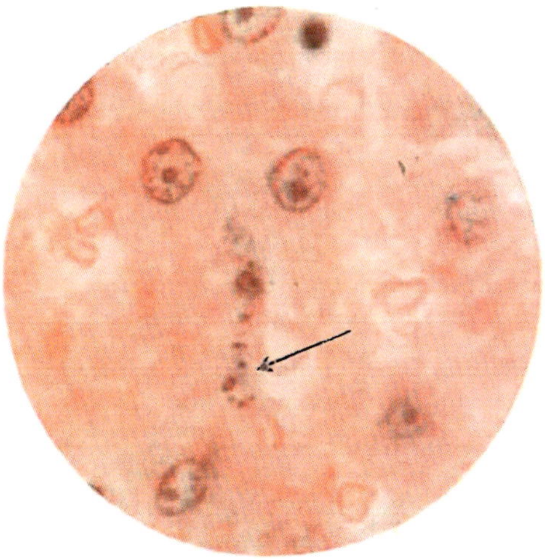

Figure 101. Bonghan sanal within the Bonghan ductule (x1,000)

This is considered to be the migration of chromatin granules into the internal Bonghan duct, ie., flow of the new-born sanal into it.

According to the examinations on vital sections of the normal liver, a single sanal starts moving actively at first in the nucleus of a resting [p96] phase and then numerous sanal follow suit in the same nucleus.

At this time, the nuclear membrane swells slightly and only moving sanal are to be seen in the nucleus.

A part of the nuclear membrane protrudes and the sanal move towards it. The bulging part expands further and finally breaks.

The sanal in the nucleus migrate into the cytoplasm through the rupture and then they come out of the cell when the cell membrane bursts.

At this time, each sanal measures about 1 micron and moves separately.

When the cells in each stage of the sanalization are fixed and stained, pictures representing the diverse conditions of the normal tissue cells as mentioned above are to be seen.

Such phenomena occurring in the normal liver tissues mean that sanal are formed in cells and they burst out of the cells, enter Bonghan ducts, and then the cells perish.

In the liver of the normal rabbit, the number of cells in the state of sanalization accounts for 2-4 per cent of the total cells.

2. Formation of cell from sanal

Nucleus-like structures are found in great numbers in the normal liver tissues; especially in the sinusoids and interlobular connective tissues. In the cell cord of the sanalizing cells are found tiny cells in the intermediate stage which are of the transitional form from round nucleus-like structures to liver cells.

Around the nuclei are recognized purple-staining cytoplasm. These cells differ from the dark cells in the pre-necrosis stage.

These are the cells either of the sole nucleus without cytoplasm or of a round nucleus-like structure with the thin layer of cytoplasm alone (Figure 102).

When the sanalization of several cells takes place simultaneously, the intensively stainable cells smaller than the liver cells, the cells with the thin layer of cytoplasm alone, the round nucleus-like structures, and the nucleus-like structures can be observed.

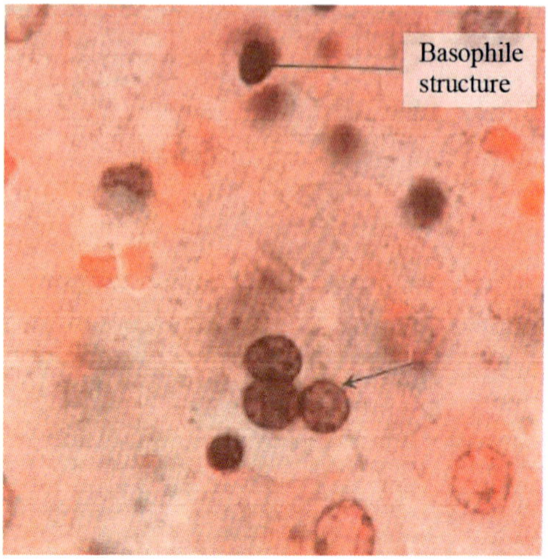

Figure 102. Nucleus-like structures in the course of the cell formation from the Bonghan sanal (x1,000)

The cells in the process of formation have no marked difference from one another, but are in a state of transition; diverse stages of gradual transition from the normal liver cell to the nucleus-like structure are recognized (Figure 103 on page 104).

In the normal liver tissues of the rabbit, the number of the cells ranging from the stage where cytoplasm is recognizable to the stage [p97] where the cells are somewhat smaller than the normal liver cells and are intensively stainable, holds 1-3 per cent of the total liver cells.

When a rabbit is starved, the number of newly-formed cells does not increase at all, whereas the number of sanalizing and perishing cells greatly increases.

In the regenerating tissues after injury, the number of cells which rupture after sanalization increases at the beginning, and later the number of the newly-formed cells increases steadily, while the number of sanalizing cells decreases. When the regeneration is complete, the number reaches the normal count.

The process of cell formation in the normal liver is the same as that from sanal in culture. In the normal liver tissues every stage of cell formation can be observed together with each stage of sanalization of nuclei. In some preparations, sanal originating from cells and going into Bonghan ducts are found. Sanal in the process of cell formation in Bonghan ducts are also to be seen in some preparations.

The circumstances that such findings are not always observed are explained by the fact that the Bonghan duct is hardly recognized in ordinary histological preparations.

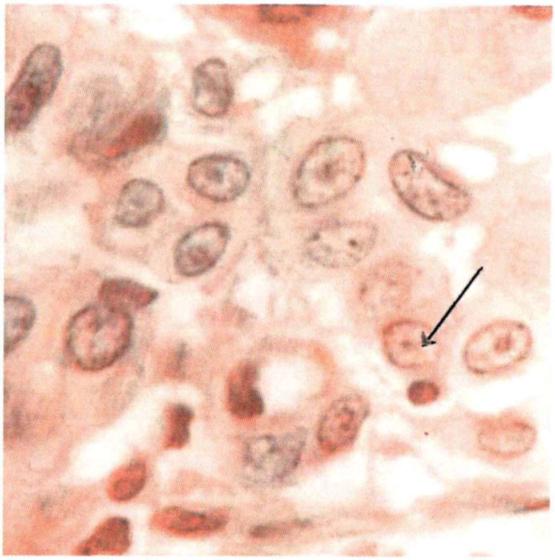

Figure 103. Immature cells formed from the Bonghan sanal (x1,000)

IV. Regeneration of injured tissues

Surmising that the "Bonghan sanal-cell cycle" would proceed actively in the organism, we studied the regeneration process of injured tissues.

A normal liver of a rabbit was injured with a glass tube, 2 mm in diameter, and histological preparations were made at different intervals.

By 12 hours after the injury occur inflammatory phenomena, i.e., haemorrhage, accumulation of leukocytes, etc. The injured liver tissue gradually changes its stainability, and turns into irregular necrosed tissue. In 24 hours after the injury, hemorrhage and accumulation of leukocytes disappear gradually and karyolysis occurs in the necrosed tissue. Then the injured cells perish entirely. In 24 hours after the injury a cluster of basophile structures measuring approximately 2-4 microns are observed around the injured area (Figure 104).

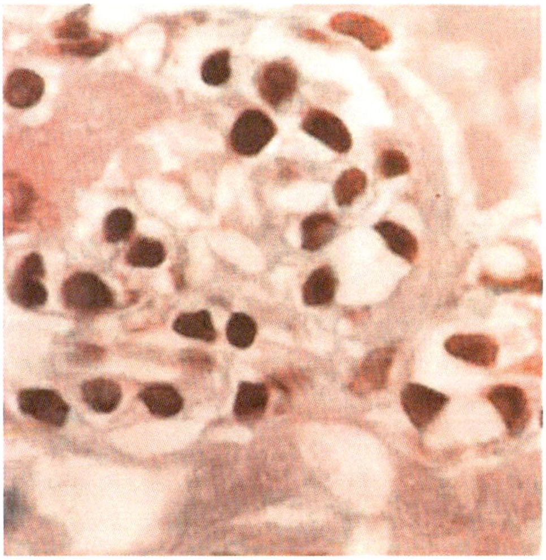

Figure 104. Basophile structures in the liver tissue 24 hours after injury (x1,000)

These basophile structures are stained deep violet by hematoxylin and show intensively positive Feulgen reaction.

These basophile structures appear abundantly in the sinusoid and [p98] interlobular connective tissues of the normal region, and gather around the injured tissue.

If sections of vital tissues separated from the injured area are observed, sanal in the stage of fusion as well as individual sanal are found moving actively. When they are fixed and stained, basophile structures are recognized.

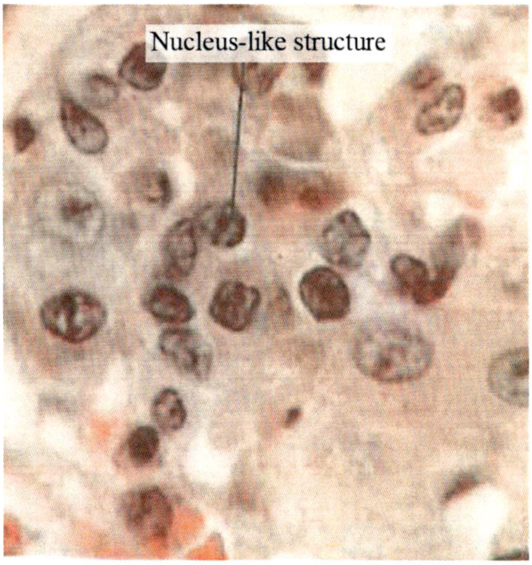

Figure 105. Liver tissue 3 days after injury (x1,000)

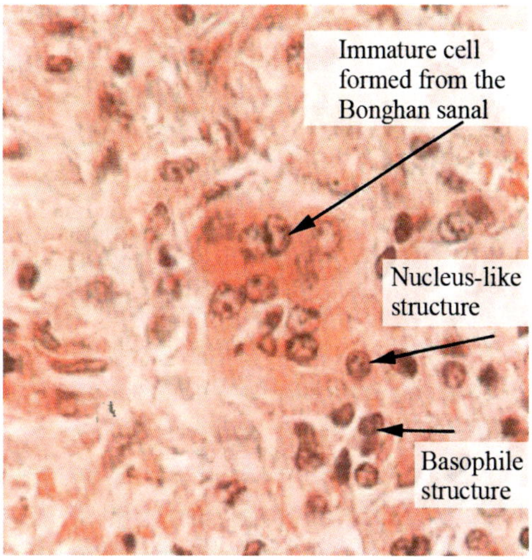

Figure 106. Part of regeneration in the liver tissue 4 days after injury (x400)

More than two days after the injury, basophile substances and lymphocyte-sized nucleus-like structures are found scattered abundantly around the central part of the affected region.

In surroundings of the injured area there appear round nucleus-like structures, around which appears the dim and thin layer of cytoplasm.

Nucleus-like structures, smaller than the nuclei of the liver cells and more intensively stainable, surround the liver cells. Such nucleus-like structures are 3-5 microns in size and become round when they grow further.

More than three days after the injury, there appear abundantly in the preparations of the injured area round nucleus-like structures and nuclei similar to those of the liver cells in the surroundings of the injured region; and nucleus-like structures are to be noted in the Bonghan duct of the sinusoid. Around the round nucleus-like structures which contain clear chromatin particles and also around the nucleus-like structures which are larger in size but less stainable than the former, appears a small amount of homogeneous cytoplasm, which is stained violet by hematoxylin-eosin (Figure 105, Figure 106, and Figure 107 on page 106).

In the vital sections at this time faint cytoplasm is to be noted around the round nucleus-like structures and it grows with the lapse of time. At the ends of the newly-formed bile ducts in the necrosed area, basophile nucleus-like structures, well stainable and without nuclear structure, are found lined up. Closely following this, cells with nuclei similar to lymphocyte and with a thin layer of cytoplasm are seen arranged, while in the other parts the cells with larger nuclei and homogeneous cytoplasm form the epithelium (Figure 108).

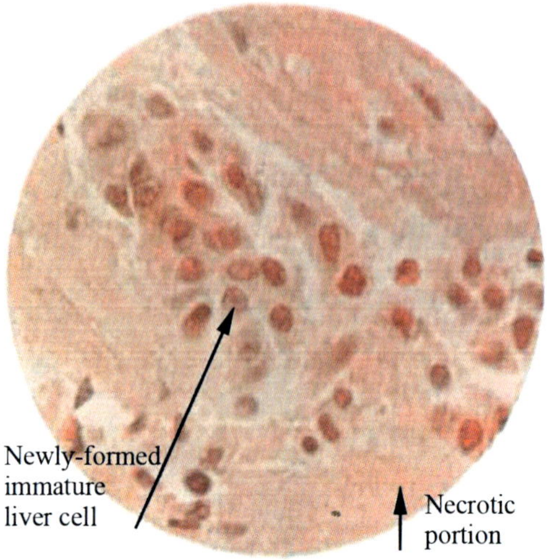

Figure 107. Liver tissue 4 days after injury (x400)

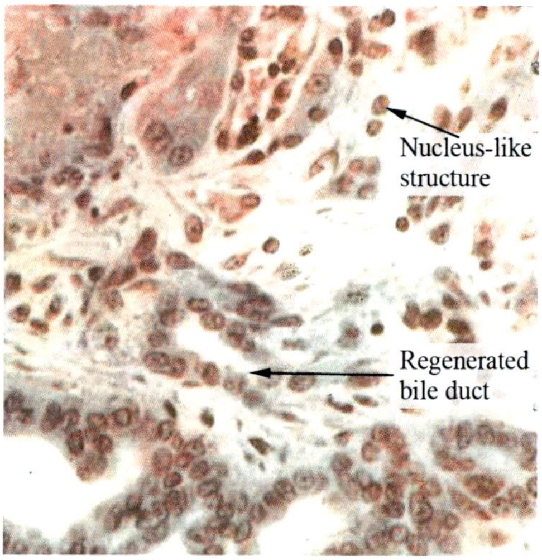

Figure 108. Regeneration process of the bile duct in the liver tissue 5 days after injury (x400)

And all the epithelial cells which have earlier formed the bile duct wall assume the shape of typical epithelial cells of the bile duct, whereas the opposite wall is formed afterwards with the cells containing nucleus similar to that of lymphocyte and these cells can not be regarded as mature epithelial cells.

About seven days after the injury, many newly-formed liver cells and small bile ducts are observed.

In the process from a nucleus-like structure to a cell, the nucleus-like structure becomes round as it matures, chromatin structures appear [p99] in it, and dim cytoplasm becomes discernible around it. When it matures further, the cytoplasm becomes more compact and is stained homogeneously purple, while the nucleus grows bigger (Figure 109).

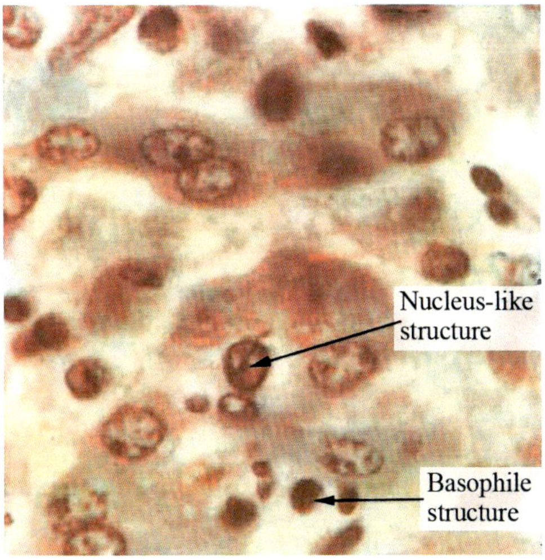

Figure 109. Liver tissue 7 days after injury (x 1,000)

Towards the end of regeneration the number of nucleus-like structures diminishes in the region of regeneration, and only mature cells are found there.

When the histological findings of cell formation in the course of regeneration after the injury of the liver are compared with findings on vital sections, the following conclusion can be made:

1) Nucleus-like structures of 3-5 microns gather around the injured area,

2) The nucleus-like structures assume spherical forms,

3) Deeply stainable cytoplasm takes shape around the round nucleus-like structures and

4) The cells mature and grow as big as normal ones (Figure 110). [p100]

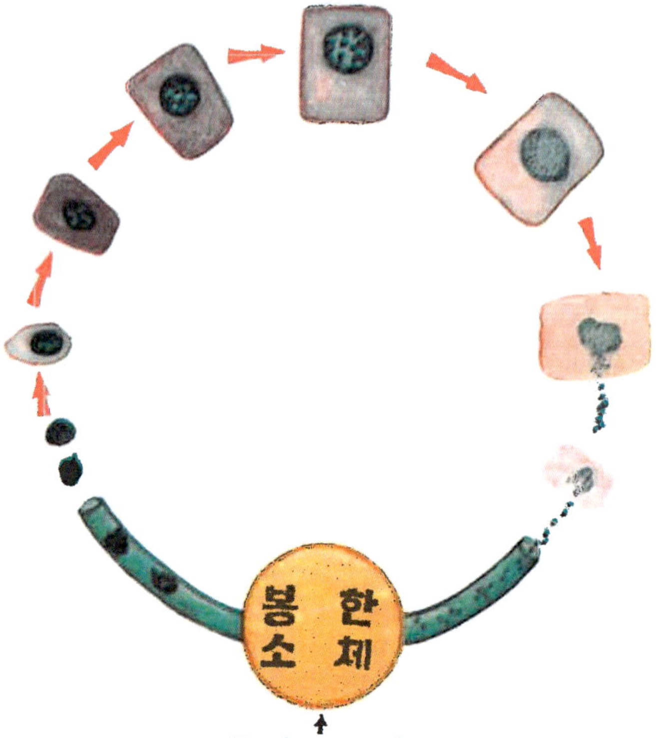

Figure 110. Diagram of the cell formation from sanal and the sanalization of cell

CONCLUSION

The afore-mentioned experimental data on sanal demonstrate the validity of the theory of sanal.

I. The self-renovation process of the organism takes the form of "Bonghan sanal-cell cycle"

A) Characteristics of Sanal

1. The form of sanal is spherical and its size measures 0.8-2.4 microns.

2. Sanal is composed of sanalosome of various forms and sanaloplasm surrounding it.

3. Sanalosome contains an abundance of DNA and sanaloplasm contains RNA.

The base composition of DNA and the mononucleotide composition of RNA are the same as those of an ordinary animal cell.

B) A sanal grows into a cell and vice versa

1. A sanal grows into a cell: a part of sanalosome protrudes and sanaloplasm appears around the process, gradually growing into a daughter sanal.

In this way, the mother sanal gives birth to many daughter sanal, which fuse and form the cell nucleus. Following the formation of the nucleus, cytoplasm takes shape around it.

2. A cell becomes scores of sanal through sanalization. Sanal formed in the cell nucleus migrate into the cytoplasm at the disappearance of the nuclear membrane.

Having entered the cytoplasm, sanal grow mature and come out of the cell, breaking the cell membrane. [p101]

C) Tissue cells are renovated through the "Bonghan sanal-cell cycle"

1. Cells are formed not only through cell division, but also from sanal.

2. The formation of cells through cell division also is a specific form of the "Bonghan sanal-cell cycle," namely, the cell division is regarded as a specific form of the processes of cell formation from sanal in which the sanalization of a cell precedes the division.

The cell division can be called a specific form of the "Bonghan sanal-cell cycle," i.e., the intracellular "Bonghan sanal-cell cycle."

3. Sanal moves incessantly on the "Bonghan sanal-cell cycle."

At each stage of this process, sanal never remains in one state, but undergoes ceaseless changes.

The state of sanal changes when they exist individually outside the cell, when they form cell nuclei after multiplication, when they lie in a resting nucleus, and finally, when a nucleus is sanalized and sanal again come out of the cell.

A sanal inside the cell nucleus has less substance of its own than the sanal outside the cell; when a sanal in the nucleus, therefore, comes out of the cell via cytoplasm, lacking substance is supplemented to it both by nucleus and cytoplasm.

4. The cell is a specific stage of the cyclic movement of sanal.

5. When cell division is proceeding, the sanalosome appears to be the so-called chromosome.

The amount of DNA contained in one sanalosome is almost equal to that of DNA in one chromosome, and when sanalization takes place within a nucleus the number of sanalosomes is equal to that of chromosomes.

The picture of the stained chromosome in the metaphase of cell division is the same as that of the sanalosome of the stained sanal.

II. All morphological constituent parts of the organism are steadily renewed

If one views the physiological renovation of tissue cells of the organism only from the angle of cell division, one's view on this subject will inevitably be too much restricted. But if the process of renovation [p102] is analysed from the standpoint of the "Bonghan sanal-cell cycle," one may learn that steady self-renovation takes place in all tissue cells. This process can also be seen clearly in sanal culture.

The steady self-renovation of the organism universally occurs not only at the molecular level but also at the cellular level. In other words, in an organism there takes place incessant metabolism as well as uninterrupted self-renovation of morphological constituents.

1) The examination of the histological preparations of normal tissues in comparison with their living specimens reveals that many processes of the "Bonghan sanal-cell cycle" go on normally and actively in the tissue cells. The sanalization of tissue cells (2-4 per cent of the cells of a rabbit liver) goes on side by side with the cell formation from sanal (1-3 per cent of the cells of a rabbit liver).

2) The process of the "Bonghan sanal-cell cycle" can be observed more clearly in the course of the regeneration of the injured tissue in which vigorous renovation takes place.

III. Self-renovation of the organism is performed by the Kyungrak system

A. Sanal exists only in the Kyungrak system

1. Sanal and different stages of its growth can be observed in all the Bonghan ducts and Bonghan corpuscles.

2. Contrary to this, almost no sanal is found in blood, lymph and tissue fluid.

3. All cells have the sanal structure and can be sanalized.

B. When a tissue cell is sanalized, sanal become mature while moving, without exception, through the circulating course of Bonghan liquor

1. When histological preparations of normal tissue cells are studied in comparison with their living specimens, it becomes clear that the sanal born of sanalization of cells enter Bonghan ducts, and while moving through them, grow into nucleus-like structures, which become cells in the relevant tissues.

2. It has been established that when sanal tagged with P32 are introduced into

Bonghan duct, they run through the circulating course of Bonghan liquor, mature in it and grow into tissue cells of organs. [p103]

3. Sanal of different stages of maturity can be seen when sanal are picked from different parts of the circulating course of Bonghan liquor.

When sanal picked out of different superficial Bonghan corpuscles are cultured, they grow into corresponding cells.

C. Bonghan liquor contains biochemical substances necessary for the growth of sanal

1. Bonghan liquor contains abundant free amino acids, free mononucleotides and hyaluronic acid, various hormones, protein, sugar and lipids.

2. Sanal grow easily into cells when they are cultivated in Bonghan liquor or in culture media of similar composition.

3. Sanal do not grow into a cell in blood, lymph or tissue fluid.

D. All the tissue cells are linked with the Kyungrak system

1. The tissue cells are directly connected with the Kyungrak system.

2. When the Bonghan duct linked with a tissue cell is cut, karyolysis occurs in the cell nucleus and the cell perishes.

The Kyungrak system regulates and controls the formation, maintenance and death of all the tissue cells.

The movements of sanal underlie all the phenomena of life.

It is considered that the basic task of biology is to delve into the law of these movements.

April 15, 1965

THE ACADEMY OF KYUNGRAK,
The Democratic People's Republic of Korea
[p104]

Also published by CuriousPages

Books by Fletcher Kovich

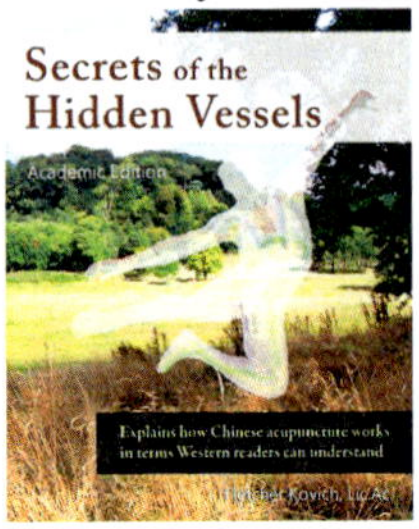

Secrets of the Hidden Vessels, Academic edition
Nonfiction. Chinese acupuncture is notoriously difficult for Western readers to understand. This book uses a new approach to clearly explain all the key aspects.

Chinese acupuncture is based on 2,000 year old Chinese scripts known as the *Nei Jing*. This book describes which parts of the *Nei Jing* are fact based, metaphorical, or untrue; identifies the conflicting *Nei Jing* theories on metabolism, and which are true or untrue; and key concepts such as the Chinese medicine organ functions are also clearly explained in relation to contemporary physiology.

The book also builds on Bong-Han Kim's work, adds much new research and uses this to provide a groundbreaking hypothesis on how acupuncture works.

The book provides students or practitioners with an indispensible guide to properly understanding the Chinese medicine of the *Nei Jing*.

Please visit **www.curiouspages.com/books** for details of free sample downloads, full details of the above books, and a complete list of books available.

Made in United States
North Haven, CT
05 November 2026

21760282R60064